Raising Mental Health Awareness in Higher Education:

Emerging Research and Opportunities

Melissa Martin
State University of New York at Plattsburgh, USA

Jean Mockry
State University of New York at Plattsburgh, USA

Alison Puliatte
State University of New York at Plattsburgh, USA

Denise A Simard
State University of New York at Plattsburgh, USA

Maureen E. Squires
State University of New York at Plattsburgh, USA

A volume in the Advances in Psychology, Mental Health, and Behavioral Studies (APMHBS) Book Series

IGI Global
DISSEMINATOR OF KNOWLEDGE

Published in the United States of America by
IGI Global
Medical Information Science Reference (an imprint of IGI Global)
701 E. Chocolate Avenue
Hershey PA, USA 17033
Tel: 717-533-8845
Fax: 717-533-8661
E-mail: cust@igi-global.com
Web site: http://www.igi-global.com

Library of Congress Cataloging-in-Publication Data

Names: Martin, Melissa, 1986- author. | Mockry, Jean, 1952- author. | Puliatte, Alison, 1975- author. | Simard, Denise A., author. | Squires, Maureen E., author.
Title: Raising mental health awareness in higher education : emerging research and opportunities / by Melissa Martin, Jean Mockry, Alison Puliatte, Denise A. Simard, and Maureen E. Squires.
Description: Hershey PA : Medical Information Science Reference, [2018] | Includes bibliographical references.
Identifiers: LCCN 2017022182| ISBN 9781522537939 (hardcover) | ISBN 9781522537946 (ebook)
Subjects: | MESH: Students--psychology | Mental Health Services | Mental Disorders--prevention & control | Universities | United States
Classification: LCC RC451.4.S7 | NLM WA 353 | DDC 616.8900835--dc23 LC record available at https://lccn.loc.gov/2017022182

This book is published in the IGI Global book series Advances in Psychology, Mental Health, and Behavioral Studies (APMHBS) (ISSN: 2475-6660; eISSN: 2475-6679)

British Cataloguing in Publication Data
A Cataloguing in Publication record for this book is available from the British Library.

All work contributed to this book is new, previously-unpublished material.
The views expressed in this book are those of the authors, but not necessarily of the publisher.

For electronic access to this publication, please contact: eresources@igi-global.com.

Advances in Psychology, Mental Health, and Behavioral Studies (APMHBS) Book Series

ISSN:2475-6660
EISSN:2475-6679

Editor-in-Chief: Bryan Christiansen, Tactical Systems, LLC, USA & Harish C. Chandan, Argosy University, USA

MISSION

The complexity of the human mind has puzzled researchers and physicians for centuries. While widely studied, the brain still remains largely misunderstood.

The **Advances in Psychology, Mental Health, and Behavioral Studies (APMHBS)** book series presents comprehensive research publications focusing on topics relating to the human psyche, cognition, psychiatric care, mental and developmental disorders, as well as human behavior and interaction. Featuring diverse and innovative research, publications within APMHBS are ideally designed for use by mental health professionals, academicians, researchers, and upper-level students.

COVERAGE

- Human Interaction
- Addiction
- Human Behavior
- Substance Abuse
- Anxiety
- Treatment & Care
- Socialization
- Mental Health & Disorders
- Neurological Disorders
- Trauma & Stress

IGI Global is currently accepting manuscripts for publication within this series. To submit a proposal for a volume in this series, please contact our Acquisition Editors at Acquisitions@igi-global.com or visit: http://www.igi-global.com/publish/.

The Advances in Psychology, Mental Health, and Behavioral Studies (APMHBS) Book Series (ISSN 2475-6660) is published by IGI Global, 701 E. Chocolate Avenue, Hershey, PA 17033-1240, USA, www.igi-global.com. This series is composed of titles available for purchase individually; each title is edited to be contextually exclusive from any other title within the series. For pricing and ordering information please visit http://www.igi-global.com/book-series/advances-psychology-mental-health-behavioral/110200. Postmaster: Send all address changes to above address.

Titles in this Series

For a list of additional titles in this series, please visit:
https://www.igi-global.com/book-series/advances-psychology-mental-health-behavioral/110200

Measuring the Psychological and Electrophysiological Attributes of Human Personality ...
Sanja Tatalović Vorkapić (University of Rijeka, Croatia)
Information Science Reference • ©2017 • 242pp • H/C (ISBN: 9781522522836) • US $130.00

Emerging Research in Play Therapy, Child Counseling, and Consltation
Rheta LeAnne Steen (Loyola University New Orleans, USA)
Information Science Reference • ©2017 • 436pp • H/C (ISBN: 9781522522249) • US $205.00

Workforce Development Theory and Practice in the Mental Health Sector
Mark Smith (Te Pou o te Whakaaro Nui: National Workforce Center for Adult Mental Health, Addiction and Disability, New Zealand) and Angela F. Jury (Te Pou o te Whakaaro Nui: National Workforce Center for Adult Mental Health, Addiction and Disability, New Zealand)
Information Science Reference • ©2017 • 378pp • H/C (ISBN: 9781522518747) • US $190.00

Improving the Quality of Life for Dementia Patients through Progressive Detection ...
Jinglong Wu (Okayama University, Japan)
Medical Information Science Reference • ©2017 • 353pp • H/C (ISBN: 9781522509257) • US $205.00

Police Psychology and Its Growing Impact on Modern Law Enforcement
Cary L. Mitchell (Pepperdine University, USA) and Edrick H. Dorian (Los Angeles Police Department, USA)
Information Science Reference • ©2017 • 345pp • H/C (ISBN: 9781522508137) • US $190.00

Seduction in Popular Culture, Psychology, and Philosophy
Constantino Martins (Nova University of Lisbon, Portugal) and Manuel Damásio (Lusófona University, Portugal)
Information Science Reference • ©2017 • 332pp • H/C (ISBN: 9781522505259) • US $175.00

For an enitre list of titles in this series, please visit:
https://www.igi-global.com/book-series/advances-psychology-mental-health-behavioral/110200

IGI Global
DISSEMINATOR OF KNOWLEDGE

701 East Chocolate Avenue, Hershey, PA 17033, USA
Tel: 717-533-8845 x100 • Fax: 717-533-8661
E-Mail: cust@igi-global.com • www.igi-global.com

Table of Contents

Preface

As educators from Institutes of Higher Education within the United States, we have all witnessed students cope with academic, social, financial, and familial struggles. However, over the course of the past decade the authors have seen a dramatic increase in the number of postsecondary students who have exhibited behaviors related to anxiety, depression, panic attacks, and suicidal ideations. Unfortunately, last year we experienced the previously unthinkable experience, one of our students committed suicide. The student was perceived as a happy go lucky student, who was a revered member of the campus community. The experience left students and faculty alike with feelings of deep sadness and wonder if this could be the destiny of the student's peers. In response, we have made a concerted effort to become better informed about matters related to the mental health, well-being, and mental illness of students on college campuses in the United States.

All authors of this book are currently faculty members in an Educator Preparation Program. Together, we have over 50 years of experience teaching in higher education in the United States. Combine that with our P-12 teaching experience and we have over one hundred years of experience in the education field. Each have noticed an increased number of teacher candidates sharing their ongoing battle with mental health issues such as anxiety, depression, panic disorders, or a general malaise. In our classes, we often ask students to reflect or share their thinking or wonderings; through this process, some of our teacher candidates have disclosed: it is hard to just get out of bed every day, let alone, thrive within a campus community; some share how they have everything they could ever want, but yet still are not happy, which makes no sense to them; they walk into a room and the first thought they have is that people are judging them negatively; they have uncontrollable mood swings that debilitate them so much they can only think of getting back to bed. They fear failure. These and the many other struggles prompted us to begin examining the trends and concerns regarding college students in the United States and mental health to see if we were part of a trend or an anomaly. It seems, we are indeed part of a growing phenomenon. The issue of college students' mental health on campuses within the U.S. is not unique to this campus.

Though our experiences are grounded in Teacher Preparation, similar experiences are not isolated within a particular area of higher education. The issues and strategies discussed here cut across programs on campuses. Staff and faculty in postsecondary institutions may find this information useful when reviewing campus policies and implementing practices that would promote student wellbeing. In the following chapters, the authors describe the current state of college student mental health in the United States, influences that contribute to non-flourishing mental health, factors (at a classroom level and campus-wide) that promote flourishing mental health, and interventions that support mental health.

In Chapter 1, "Introduction: Mental Health and Well-Being of College Students," the authors examine the transition from high to college. For many students, the transition to college means a faster pace, heavier academic workload, financial burden, competition, and new social situations. The aspects of the transition can be exhilarating or they can create circumstances whereby college students languish or experience negative mental health. The authors seek to provide an overview of trends, influences, needs, and supports for postsecondary students with mental health concerns.

In Chapter 2, "Mental Health and Well-Being: Societal Influences," the authors discuss factors that shape college students' mental health status. In particular, they focus on two major influences, social construct and the impact of family. Social construct includes economics and status, and technology (as these students are seen as digital natives), and affiliation as a member of an underrepresented group that isolates rather than builds a collaborative, healthy membership in the larger community. Family pertains to parenting that obstructs the development of life skills for success, creating frustrations, anxieties and unrealistic expectations that diminishes their confidence to persevere, problem solve and contribute to society.

In Chapter 3, "Dispositional Factors Influencing College Success: Personality, Character, and Mindset," the authors examine personality traits that may help students overcome challenges or stress in college. Specifically, grit, self-control, resiliency, and self-compassion are explored in terms of success in college. The authors posit that these traits are also essential when these students become general and special education teachers in public and private K-12 schools. Furthermore, this chapter explores fixed versus growth mindsets and how that construct can also influence student success (and thus well-being) while enrolled in coursework.

In Chapter 4, "Strategies for the College Classroom," the authors explore a model of emotional intelligence that describes how emotions are processed. They then discuss how our ability to regulate our emotions impacts our social interactions. Next, mindfulness based practices is presented as an approach to develop effective emotional regulation. Finally, a review of mindfulness based practices that can be incorporated into a college classroom is presented.

In Chapter 5, "Campus-Wide Initiatives," the authors situate mental health issues in the context of U.S. institutes of higher education. They provide a brief history of the provision of mental health services on campus and contends that postsecondary schools should shift to a campus-wide, preventive, proactive approach to promote student flourishing. Four specific areas for interventions are discussed. These include academic or curricular adjustments, increased awareness and knowledge, supportive environments, and appropriate policies and procedures. These initiatives (which are not only the responsibility of "experts") rely on the open communication and collaboration of all members of the campus community.

In Chapter 6, What Is Next? Future Considerations," the authors present programs and activities that they will propose to be implemented in their current setting. In addition, the authors present a possible research study examining relationships between personality traits and perceived mental health of current college students. The goal of the study is to develop college coursework and support programs to address the unique needs of the authors' students.

Chapter 1
Introduction:
Mental Health and Well-Being of College Students

Denise Simard
State University of New York at Plattsburgh, USA

Melissa Martin
State University of New York at Plattsburgh, USA

Jean Mockry
State University of New York at Plattsburgh, USA

Alison Puliatte
State University of New York at Plattsburgh, USA

Maureen E. Squires
State University of New York at Plattsburgh, USA

ABSTRACT

As educators, the authors have all witnessed students cope with academic, social, financial, and familial struggles. However, there seems to be a growing trend whereby they are witnessing students who are feeling an increasing sense of hopeless and inability to persist. Students appear to lack competence, grit, or resilience to work through adversity. This chapter helps readers contextualize the challenges students are facing and how faculty members are gaining the knowledge and skills to learn and understand mental illness, mental health, and well-being in order to improve their ability to serve, support, and educate.

DOI: 10.4018/978-1-5225-3793-9.ch001

INTRODUCTION

As educators, we have all witnessed students cope with academic, social, financial, and familial struggles. However, there seems to be a growing trend whereby we are witnessing students who are feeling an increasing sense of hopeless and inability to persist. Students appear to lack competence, grit, or resilience to work through adversity. Our students frequently express to us how difficult it is: to simply get out of bed in the morning to face the day; focus on school work; cope with the stresses of family; maintain (or leave) relationships; eat; sleep; exercise; enjoy the things they once loved. In the words of one student (who shall remain anonymous for obvious reasons), "I am unsure of my future and that scares me. I am lethargic, unmotivated and very comfortable. Real talk, my grades are dropping because of these things. Okay, so how am I going to change myself, my habits?" These comments and experiences of our students have led us to take a deep dive into the research to better understand the trends, influences, needs, mindsets, strategies for success, campus-wide initiatives, and supports for postsecondary students with mental health concerns.

As faculty members we serve as instructors, advisors, mentors, and confidants. One of the real challenges we face is effectively identifying and supporting students who are struggling with negative mental health. The college students who may be in the greatest need of supports or connectedness may well be those students who are not showing up socially or emotionally prepared to engage within the college community. It is sometimes extremely difficult know who these students are, they often are able to present themselves very well, even though there are struggles deep within. Frequently, our first warning signs include students missing classes, advisement, or other scheduled events (and not notifying someone), or students who were once active become withdrawn or isolate themselves from peers or activities they love, or when students are physically present but not active participants. Typically, students do not immediately self-disclose their struggles for fear of being judged or other possible negative stigmas they may perceive.

When we are fortunate enough to have students self-disclose, we frequently feel underprepared to support them. Due in large part because our professional preparation does not explicitly address the role we have assumed as a potential first responder to a students' mental health or well-being. As faculty, our typical responses include to listen, refer students to on-campus or community health care or academic support services, provide extended time to complete assignments, pre-plan for anxiety producing events, discuss ways to take breaks and de-stress, facilitate family meetings, host weekly check-ins, or just be present. While these approaches may provide some with a sense of belonging or support in the short-term, we have anecdotally not deemed our efforts as being successful in providing a means for students to develop increased sustained coping skills, resiliency, or grit. According to Douce and Keeling (2014), "A resilient person copes with trouble or trauma and bounces back. Resilience protects psychological well-being and is an indicator of its presence." (p. 2). Given many of our students face challenges, and are not successful in "bouncing back," we are seeking to improve our ability to serve, support, and educate. It seems we have discovered mental health and well-being have the potential to create pervasive challenges for students with regard to the classroom, community, relationships, self-esteem, motivation, and hope.

MENTAL HEALTH AND WELL-BEING

In order to understand the two continuums models of mental health and well-being and mental illness, we must examine their definitions more closely. The Center for Disease Control (2016) indicates, "Mental illnesses refer to disorders generally characterized by dysregulation of mood, thought, and/ or behavior." The Medline Plus Medical Dictionary (n. d.) further defines mental illness as, "any of a broad range of medical conditions (such as major depression, schizophrenia, obsessive compulsive disorder, or panic disorder) that are marked primarily by sufficient disorganization of personality, mind, or emotions to impair normal psychological functioning and cause marked distress or disability and that are typically associated with a disruption in normal thinking, feeling, mood, behavior, interpersonal interactions, or daily functioning." According to the World Health Organization (WHO, 2014), "Mental health is defined as a state of well-being in which every individual realizes his or her own potential, can cope with the normal stresses of life, can work productively and fruitfully, and is able to make a contribution to her or his community." Keyes and Westerhof (2010) state, "Mental health has long been defined as the absence of psychopathologies, such as depression and anxiety." (p. 110). Even though the definitions of the terms are very different, the absence of a mental illness does not represent mental health. In her influential work, Jahoda (1958) clearly stated "...the absence of mental illness is not a sufficient indicator of mental health." (p. 15). Making these distinctions and knowing the differences are important for us as faculty members to consider and keep in mind as students show up in our offices, classrooms, and campuses. Our responses and support may require increased communication with our colleagues in student affairs (e.g. residence life, student health center, student psychological center) and professionals and community-based organizations (e.g. National Alliance on Mental Illness, Alcoholics Anonymous, Behavioral/Health Centers, Health Department, Al-Anon).

In order to more thoroughly understand mental health, one needs to examine components of the definition put forth by the WHO (2014). While the definition put forth by WHO (2014) is widely accepted, some feel it limits the scope of the reference of mental health only to subjective emotional well-being. The United States Department of Health and Human Services (n. d.) seeks to expand the definition, "Mental health includes our emotional, psychological, and social well-being." These components provide a means to examine well-being in more functional and meaningful ways than the dichotomous thinking of mental illness or mental health and well-being. It allows for the utilization of a continuum model from which to examine mental illness and mental health and well-being.

The WHO (2014) definition of mental health is identified as a state of well-being, but what is well-being? The term is considered subjective by many. Ryan and Deci (2001) specify that well-being, is a conceptualization of the optimal functioning and experiences of individuals. This concept of well-being is based upon two distinct philosophies: hedonia and eudaimonia. Huta (2015) indicates that it is necessary to study both hedonia and eudaimonia well-being and their distinctions in order to fully operationalize and comprehend the continuum of languishing and flourishing. Just as mental health and mental illness are neither equal nor opposite, the same is true for hedonia and eudaimonia. Huta (2015) indicates they "... are not opposites, nor are they mutually exclusive – they are complementary psychological functions." (p.3).

The deliberations around hedonia and Eudaimonia is not a new one. In fact, Huta (2016) indicates the distinction between hedonia and eudaimonia dates back more than 2500 years! Keyes, Shmotkin, and Ryff, (2002) point out the hedonic and eudaimonic theoretical perspectives of well-being attend to that which makes people feel good or happy and function well. Keyes (2013, p. 6) states, "The hedonic tradition is reflected in the stream of research on subjective emotional well-being (i.e. happiness, satisfaction, and affect balance)." In their research Huta and Waterman (2014) have determined eudaimonia theoretical constructs tend to emphasize concepts such as pursuit of self-actualization, growth mindset, balance needs of self and others, consider abstract and bigger picture concerns, engage in ethical and moral actions, and focus on present and future. Keyes (2013, p.6) further asserts eudaimonia, "…reflects how well individuals see themselves functioning in life, striving to achieve secular standards of excellence, such as purpose, contribution, integration, intimacy, acceptance, and mastery." In short, Huta and Ryan (2010) have described hedonia as seeking personal well-being and eudaimonia as typically striving to achieve personal well-being and supporting or facilitating the well-being in others as well.

Deiner (1984) points out that until late in the 20th century the emphasis in the field of psychology emphasized unhappiness and suffering. Prior, there was little consideration given to happiness and positive well-being, or more specifically the concept of flourishing. The use of a two-continuum model allows for a means to examine gradations or progressions for such things as mental health, well-being, and mental illness. Keyes (2002) states, "The mental health continuum consists of complete and incomplete mental health. Adults with complete mental health are flourishing in life with high levels of well-being." (p. 210). He goes on to say, "Adults with incomplete mental health are languishing in life with low well-being." (p. 210). The investigation of the theory of flourishing requires a deeper examination and understanding of the pursuit of happiness and its impact on well-being.

As pointed out, hedonic perspectives reflect emotional well-being. Eudaimonic perspectives on the other hand represent psychological well-being and social well-being (Ryff, 1989; Keyes, 2002). Keyes (2013) reports emotional well-being is more subjective than psychological well-being. This is true because emotional well-being is based upon perceptions of happiness, satisfaction, positive and negative effects. Keyes (2013) clarifies happiness further by indicating is measurement is predicated on spontaneous reactions or responses to an instant experience versus a long-term evaluation which better signifies overall life satisfaction. Fink (2014, p. 381) distinguishes emotional and psychological well-being as follows, "An individual described as exhibiting psychological well-being finds meaning and purposeful direction in life, accepts self, seeks continued personal development, acts, and thinks autonomously, and can establish positive relationships with others." Keyes (2002) asserts the positive sense of meaning from social interactions, connections, relationships, sense of belonging, and interest in the greater good of society represents an individual's social well-being. Douce and Keeling (2014) add, "A key component of well-being is resilience—the ability to recognize, face, and manage or overcome problems and challenges, and to be strengthened, rather than defeated, in the process." (p. 2)

In further distinguishing emotional and psychological well-being, Keyes (2013, pp. 7-8) states, "In contrast to the subjective measures of well-being, psychological well-being requires individuals to self-report about the quality with which they are functioning in their lives (not feelings or emotions toward or about life)." According to Keyes (2002, p. 208), "Positive functioning consists of six dimensions of psychological well-being: self-acceptance, positive relations with others, personal growth, purpose in life, environmental mastery, and autonomy." These dimensions are important aspects to examining levels of well-being. Ryan and Deci (2001) maintain eudaimonic theories may produce desired outcomes which are pleasurable, but they may not necessarily be positive or good for an individual and would therefore not promote positive well-being.

PERVASIVE PROBLEM

American K-12 schools and college campuses are facing increases in negative mental health and incomplete well-being at alarming rates across America. In particular, there are high numbers of children and youth who experience psychological stress. Over the past several years, we have seen evidence of patterns of negative mental health and incomplete well-being for students in both our undergraduate and graduate teacher education programs; however, we recognize these struggles and psychological stress began prior to college admission. According to The Child Mind Institute (CMI) (2016), 20% of America's children would meet the criteria to be diagnosed with a major mental disorder. They also indicate, 80% of chronic mental disorders start during childhood. Furthermore, CMI (2016, p. 2) states, "Fifty percent of mental health disorders begin before age 14 and 75% before age 24, affecting the learning and school experience for all children." The National Alliance on Mental Illness (NAMI) (2014) points out there is typically an 8-10-year delay between the onset of the mental health disorder and the intervention. This is a critical insight for those of us who work with students who tend to be between 18 and 24 years of age. These data represent and alarming epidemic, regarding the mental health and well-being of America's children and youth.

Graduating from high school and entering college often represents one of the first major transitions in the lives of America's youth. The trend for college enrollment has grown since the beginning of the 21st Century. According to the United States Department of Education, National Center for Educational Statistics (NCES) (2016a) since fall 2000, college enrollments have increased by 5.2 million. They estimate 20.5 million students enrolled in American Colleges and Universities in fall 2016. In examining demographic data related to the "traditional" college student, a student between 18 and 24, the NCES (2016a) indicate approximately 85% are undergraduate students, 57% are females 14.5% are Black and 34.7% are Hispanic.

Levens, Elrahal and Sagui (2016) declare that one theory why freshman college students struggle with mental health and well-being is due in large part to the fact for many, college requires their lives to be uprooted and they must learn to live in a new community, on their own. Such life events create sweeping changes and often result in increased levels of stress and negative consequences. Gruttado and Crudo (2012) state these negative outcomes regarding well-being can have a direct impact on an individual student's retention, persistence, and academic success in college as well as those around them (e.g. family, friends, roommates). These findings confirm much of the experiences and psychological stress our college students have shared with us as they navigate critical transitions from high school to college, undergraduate programs to graduate programs, and college to careers.

Regardless of gender, the transition to college poses significant challenges related to mental health and well-being. Unfortunately, it is quite common for both males and females to experience negative mental health while enrolled in degree programs on a college campus. In their study regarding psychosocial adjustment, Conley et al. (2014, p. 205) determined males and females experience comparable sharp declines throughout their first semester on campus. However, the distress for males tends to plateau around the middle of the first year; however, female distress continues to get worse throughout the year. This trend is consistent with research which has found females tend to internalize distress more than males, and potentially experience greater issues related to body issues, body part and facial feature comparisons, and eating disorders (Conley and Rudolph, 2009; Malinauskas, et al., 2006). Ridner et al. (2015) determined heterosexual students express greater levels of well-being than do members of the gay, lesbian, bisexual, transsexual, or questioning community, the higher the students' GPA, the better the mean level of well-being, and it seemed the strongest predictor of well-being is sleep quality (pp. 119-120).

While both males and females experience a continuum of mental health and well-being, there are a few distinctions. Conley et al. (2014, p. 195) point out:

Examining gender differences in developmental trajectories revealed that females experience additional elevations in psychological distress even after the immediate transition, while males evidenced worse baseline levels in cognitive-affective vulnerabilities, cognitive-affective strengths, and social well-being.

This is of particular concern since the U. S. Department of Education (2012) determined females earn over 60 percent of associate's degrees and approximately 57 percent of bachelor's degrees. This is of particular importance to us due to the fact that in our department most of the students we currently work with are white middle class women. Therefore, when providing supports during the first year of college for students, we need to be more cognizant of the need to provide sustained efforts for our female students.

UNIQUE ENVIRONMENT AND INFLUENCES

Attending college affords individuals numerous opportunities to grow and learn. According the PEW Research Center (2011) the purposes for attending college in the United States include personal and intellectual growth, a means to learn work-related knowledge and skills, or a combination therein. It seems however, there are aspects beyond academics in which many must grapple with. While college can bring lots of excitement and opportunities, it is also frequently met with great distress. According to the American College Health Association's (ACHA) National College Health Assessment II (NCHA) (2016) 17% of student respondents reported having been treated by a professional for anxiety, 13.9% for depression and 8.4% for panic disorders. Furthermore, data from the ACHA (2016) indicate that students most frequently identified stress, sleep difficulties, and anxiety as barriers to academic success.

Data from the ACHA (2016) show for college student respondents in the United States: 36.7% felt so depressed that it was difficult to function; 58.4% felt overwhelming anxiety; 9.8% seriously considered suicide; 6.7% intentionally cut, burned, bruised, or otherwise injured yourself; 39.6% felt overwhelming anger; 65% felt very sad; 49.8% felt things were hopeless; 85.1% felt overwhelmed by all you had to do; 81.7% felt exhausted (not from physical activity); and 59.3% felt very lonely, any time within the last 12 months. Keyes (2002, p. 210) states, "The mental health continuum consists of complete and incomplete mental health. Adults with complete mental health are flourishing in life with high levels of well-being." This statement indicates an individual has positive emotion and is functioning well socially and psychologically. Conversely, individuals with low well-being, or who feel loneliness, emptiness, hopelessness, worthlessness, or stagnation are languishing.

A college campus is rather unique. Eisenberg, Golberstein, and Hunt (2009) point out college campuses are interconnected on multiple levels given students live, learn, and interact socially within the same environment. Eisenberg, Golberstein, Hunt (2009) further highlight the existence of anxiety, depression, and panic attacks all impact the capacity of college students to persist and to be successful socially and academically. In our experiences in working with college students who regularly communicate an overall malaise regarding their overall well-being; finding motivation to get out of bed let alone be physically active can seem like a Herculean task. For students who are not physically or socially active, the transition to college is one in which often results in "…steep declines in psychological well-being, cognitive-affective strengths, and social well-being as well as increases in psychological distress and cognitive-affective vulnerabilities." (Conley et al., 2014, p. 195). Keyes (2002) notes when an individual is languishing, there is a high likelihood of absences for school or work. This is of particular concern for college students. Missing classes and falling behind can exacerbate already languishing mental health and make it more difficult for faculty and staff to provide support. Keyes (2002) indicates depressive episodes can create similar lost work or school attendance, and individuals who have co-morbid episodes of languishing and depression have significantly worse levels of functioning.

Levens, Elrahal and Sagui (2016) stress a strong predictor of positive mental health and well-being for college students is the student's support network. Unfortunately, however the American College Health Association (2012) asserts many college students experience challenges in remaining physically and socially active. The ACHA (2012) finding is of particular importance because as researchers such as Maher et al. (2012) indicate when individuals regularly engage in physical and social activities, the individual live a healthier lifestyle and experience improved mental health and well-being. The outcomes of research by Ridner et al. (2015) further supports such claims: students with lower BMI's, and were physically active, slept well, or those who did not use tobacco or illicit drugs expressed greater well-being (p. 119). These findings are affirmed in the following messaged received from a student prior to an advising session,

This semester conveniently aligns with perhaps the first, of many I assume, short period of times in my life where I don't feel equipped or capable of doing what I have to do. Recently, I've been emotionally distancing myself from school, from the gym, really any healthy habits have seemed to get just a little further away. This semester I've drank heavily, smoked illicit substances, and stayed up later than I should most nights. I slept past my morning science class one to[sic] many times and my professor advised me not to come in anymore. (Anonymous, 2017, p. 1)

While most students do not as clearly articulate their struggles, many face these challenges and are unable to persevere.

In addition to physical and social activities, families play an important role in the positive mental health and well-being of college students. Rohmer and Britner (2002) determined there is a connection between parental acceptance and overall psychological well-being, hedonia and eudaimonia, and low psychological suffering. Another parental factor is emotional support. It is more common than one would expect to have a parent call us as faculty members and seek to "fix" a concern. Parents may work collaboratively (or sometimes not so collaboratively) to resolve an issue of behalf of their child-regardless of the circumstances surrounding the particular issue or concern. The issues could be anything from a grade grievance, roommate issue, scheduling conflict. Frequently, when advocating for their child, it has been our experience that little mention or consideration is given to student accountability or responsibility around the specific matter. While these calls are intended to be helpful to students, there is evidence that such parental behaviors can be detrimental to the ability of their child to develop resiliency or experience positive mental health or well-being. Levens, Elrahal and Sagui (2016) found when students were provided with emotional support from parents, students were more successful in developing effective coping skills than when instrumental supports such as money or a car were provided by parents. The emotional support appears to facilitate greater positive mental health and well-being.

There seems to be significant evidence that family relationships impact the well-being and mental health of children and youth. Ross, Hood, and Short (2016, p. 372) point out, "The family unit is the first socialization a child experiences and perceptions of these familial experiences can shape our working models of relationships, including beliefs, and expectations." When children experience chaos and unpredictability, they may develop an unpredictability belief system. Ross and Hill (2002, p. 458) formally described the unpredictability schema as "…a pervasive belief that people are undependable and the world is chaotic." Ross and McDuff (2008) state some factors unpredictability may include economic struggles, separation or divorce, family member with depression or anxiety, and crime rate within neighborhood. Ross, Short, and Garofano (2016) note unpredictability within the family unit correlates to the development of fundamentally flawed belief systems of uncertainty and lower self-efficacy, which can have negative impacts on mental health and well-being.

BARRIERS TO SEEKING PROFESSIONAL SUPPORT

Students with mental health issues cannot receive services without disclosing their disorder. However, many students often refrain from self-disclosure. National Alliance on Mental Illness (NAMI) (2012), found the top reason students do not disclose are: "Fear or concern for the impact disclosing would have on how students, faculty and staff perceive them, including within mental health degree programs." (p. 9). These reasons illustrate how real the worry is for some students regarding the perceived stigma negative mental health can carry. This may also demonstrate a desire not to be seen as an outsider or different from others. Ultimately such fear limits access and potentially overall psychological well-being.

College campuses seek to support students who may be languishing; however, many students do not seek services for a variety of reasons. Goguen et al. (2016, p. 45) points out, "Barriers to seeking treatment may stem from fear of public stigma (that the individual will be perceived or treated negatively by others), self-stigma (that the person will feel less confident or good about themselves), or feelings of shame." Some of our college students confirm the existence of these barriers, they are often still trying to "fit in" and seeking help for a mental health concern can exacerbate the challenges of transitioning into a new environment and perpetuate negative perceptions of self. So in lieu of seeking professional supports our students tend to either remain silent about their languishing, resort to maladaptive behaviors (alcohol or illicit drugs), rely on the support of friends/roommates and family members. We do feel compelled to share that anecdotally speaking, we are seeing an increase in the number of students who are self-disclosing their languishing behaviors or personal mental health histories.

There appears to be a gender disparity regarding the recognition and disclosure of psychological distress. Furnham, Cook, and Batey (2011) point out male students frequently do not identify their languishing behaviors or mental health struggles. Furthermore, they indicate when males are aware of their spiraling mental health they are less likely to seek support due to an increased perception of stigma regarding mental health and the need for professional help or supports. Sometimes the hesitancy comes from a lack of awareness that there is a problem, that they are languishing. Other times, they are unaware of potential supports and services. Many college students come to our offices indicating they have support team at home, but they have not yet established a treatment team on campus or in the local community around campus. Other students also share that their problems do not appear as significant as those of their peers and will allow a peer to access limited campus services in lieu of seeking the support.

We know college students often seek help informally. Eisenberg et al. (2011) determined 78% of student respondents with negative mental health sought support from nonprofessionals such as family members (52%) and friends (67%). We also know support networks are predictors of positive or mental health. However, it is risky for a college student to rely solely upon the support of peers while languishing. Family and peers often do not feel prepared to take on the responsibilities of a mental health professional. For example, Davies, Wardlaw, Morriss, and Glazebrook (2016, p. 7) found, 64% of peers would provide information and support for a fellow student; however, only 13% felt very confident about helping a student with symptoms of depression and 40% expressed either no or only slight confidence in their ability to do so.

An additional challenge underrepresented populations have to consider when seeking support for a mental health concern is the cultural competence of the provider. This is a significant concern given NAMI (2015b) has indicated 28.3% of American Indians/Alaska Native, 19.3% of white, 18.6% of Black, 16.3% of Hispanic, and 13.9% of Asian adults live with a mental health condition. It is critical for us to be aware of current and shifting demographics, and the impact on mental health. NAMI (2015a, p. 1) states, "African Americans are 20% more likely to experience serious psychological distress than White Americans." Individuals from the LGBTQ community are two times as likely to have a mental health condition as their heterosexual counterparts (NAMI, 2015b, p. 2). NAMI (2015b) indicates, "11% of transgender individuals reported being denied care by mental health clinics due to bias or discrimination." (p. 2). According to NAMI (2015a), "Cultural biases against mental health and health care professionals in general prevent many African Americans from accessing care due to prior experiences with historical misdiagnoses, inadequate treatment and a lack of cultural understanding." (p. 1).

Some additional challenges students with mental health concerns face is the possibility of faculty feeling uncomfortable talking about or working with students to find appropriate accommodations. This may in part be due to the fact, most faculty have been prepared with content knowledge within a particular discipline, but not how to address the unique needs of college students with mental health concerns. Condra et al. (2015, p. 284) state, "… many faculty reported that they felt uncomfortable interacting with these students." Milligan (2010) asserts much of the discomfort and negative attitudes come due to a lack of awareness regarding appropriate accommodations and supports for students who have negative mental health. Faculty are in a precarious position, most of us are hired under the impression our primary responsibility is to support student academic learning. However, the reality is, that is a small portion of the role. Once faculty form relationships with students, they tend to share deeply personal and often painful details of their personal lives. It is in the moment when students share their lived experiences and subsequent psychological distress we feel the reality of our under preparedness to support students as they navigate the labyrinth of life often filled with loneliness, loss, trauma, despair, stress, anxiety, depression, and suicidal ideations.

CAMPUS-WIDE INITITATIVES AND SUPPORTS

Siggins (2010, p. 146) points out the important for student well-being to be a campus-wide concern, not merely the purview of the campus psychological health centers, "the whole community must be responsible for the provision of care to the student." Furthermore, Douce and Keeling (2014, p. 6) advocate for, "Eliminating fragmentation and improving access in supporting students' health, well-being, and learning" with the purpose of developing a campus culture whereby student well-being is deeply embedded into the mission of every college campus. In the National Alliance on Mental Illness (NAMI) (2012) report, College Students Speak: A Survey Report on Mental Health, key findings and suggestions were made. Students surveyed felt in addition to campus counseling services and supports, integrating drug and alcohol and mental health programs and mental health training for the entire campus community were essential services and supports. Furthermore, the NAMI (2012) study revealed the top 5 reasons students found colleges supportive (with regard to mental health) number 2 on the list was, "The school understands that college can be stressful and that mental health is a priority. The college educates faculty, staff and students on mental health." (p. 19). In contrast, the primary reason students found colleges not supportive (with regard to mental health) includes, "The school does not educate faculty, staff and students on mental health. Thus, stigma persists and professors do not follow accommodations." (p. 19). The second reason was, "They do not publicly acknowledge or discuss mental health issues with the campus community and the impact these issues can have on students." (NAMI, 2012, p. 19). Corroborating the perceived need for professional development is the 79% of respondents who indicate mental health training for faculty and staff, it was identified as the single most important awareness activity colleges can provide! Connecting the academic and student supports on college campuses may provide a more comprehensive support system for all.

Douce and Keeling (2014) call for a shift in attitudes concerning mental health and well-being on college campuses, to challenge current perceptions and stereotypes and empower more students to access services and engage in activities to promote flourishing well-being. They indicate one goal college campuses should strive to attain is: "Nurturing a supportive tone and attitude about mental health in campus culture to challenge stereotypes about mental health problems, undermine prejudices and stigma about counseling, and provide encouragement to students to reflect on their own mental health and seek services when needed." (p. 7). Morales (2014) suggest in order to support students in developing resiliency, college campus must support students' developing strong self-efficacy skills; assist students in realistically examining their strengths and weaknesses; and promoting better help seeking behaviors. (p. 192). Such a shift that would provide opportunities for college faculty to learn and develop skills needed to assist students in being more resilient and create a more inclusive culture.

CONCLUSION

As we embarked upon this endeavor, we ourselves were unaware of many of the available programs and supports available. We embrace the goal put forth by Douce and Keeling (2014) which states, "Providing outreach education and consultation to prepare all members of the campus community to recognize and respond to students with mental or behavioral health concerns." (p.7). Much of the training provided on college campuses focuses on the Student

Affairs personnel (understandably so); however, faculty see students on a regular basis (and if we do not see a student over time, red flags are raised), we serve as mentors, academic advisors, advisors for clubs, sororities and fraternities, all of which require direct interaction with students. Engaging faculty in campus-wide initiatives may create mechanisms for earlier alerts to languishing behaviors or negative mental health. We strongly advocate for greater involvement in campus initiatives which can lead to increased accommodations and supports. We hope our journey and lessons learned help you better support young adults within postsecondary education programs.

REFERENCES

American College Health Association. (2012). *American College Health Association-National College Health Assessment II: Reference Group Executive Summary Spring 2012*. Hanover, MD: American College Health Association.

American College Health Association. (2016). *American College Health Association-National College Health Assessment II: Reference Group Executive Summary Spring 2016*. Hanover, MD: American College Health Association.

Center for Disease Control. (2016, August 11). Mental Illness. Retrieved March 14, 2017, from https://www.cdc.gov/mentalhealth/basics/mental-illness.htm

Child Mind Institute. (2016). Children's Mental Health Report. Retrieved March 25, 2017 from https://childmind.org/report/2016-childrens-mental-health-report/

Condra, M., Dineen, M., Gills, H., Jack-Davies, A., & Condra, E. (2015). Academic accommodations for postsecondary students with mental health disabilities in Ontario, Canada: A review of the literature and reflections on emerging issues. *Journal of Postsecondary Education and Disability*, *28*(3), 277–291.

Conley, C. S., & Rudolph, K. D. (2009). The emerging sex difference in adolescent depression: Interacting contributions of puberty and peer distress. *Development and Psychopathology*, *21*(02), 593–620. doi:10.1017/S0954579409000327 PMID:19338700

Conley, S. C., Kirsch, C. A., Dickson, A. D., & Bryant, B. F. (2014). Negotiating the transition to college: Developmental trajectories and gender differences in psychological functioning, cognitive affective strategies, and social well-being. *Emerging Adulthood 2(3),* 195-210. Retrieved April 3, 2017 from: http://journals.sagepub.com/doi/pdf/10.1177/2167696814521808

Davies, E. B., Wardlaw, J., Morriss, R., & Glazebrook, C. (2016). An experimental study exploring the impact of vignette gender on the quality of university students' mental health first aid for peers with symptoms of depression. *BMC Public Health, 16*(1), 1–11. doi:10.1186/s12889-016-2887-2 PMID:26911725

Diener, E. (1984). Subjective well-being. *Psychological Bulletin, 95*(3), 542–575. doi:10.1037/0033-2909.95.3.542 PMID:6399758

Douce, L. A., & Keeling, R. P. (2014). A strategic primer on college student mental health. Retrieved April 8, 2017 from https://www.naspa.org/images/uploads/main/Campus_Mental_Health_Primer_web_final.pdf

Eisenberg, D., Golberstein, E., & Hunt, J. (2009). Mental health and academic success in college. *The B.E. Journal of Economic Analysis & Policy, 9*(1), 40. doi:10.2202/1935-1682.2191

Eisenberg, D., Hunt, J., Speer, N., & Zivin, K. (2011). Mental health service utilization among college students in the United States. *The Journal of Nervous and Mental Disease, 199*(5), 301–308. doi:10.1097/NMD.0b013e3182175123 PMID:21543948

Furnham, A., Cook, R., & Batey, M. (2011). Mental health literacy among university students. *Journal of Mental Health (Abingdon, England), 10*(4), 198–210.

Goguen, K., Britt, T., Jennings, K., Sytine, A., Jeffirs, S., Peasley, A., & Palmer, J. et al. (2016). Implicit and explicit attitudes towards mental health treatment. *Journal of Social and Clinical Psychology, 35*(1), 45–63. doi:10.1521/jscp.2016.35.1.45

Gruttadaro, D., & Crudo, D. (2012). College students speak: A survey report on mental 125 health. Retrieved April 8, 2017 from https://www.nami.org/getattachment/About-NAMI/Publications-Reports/Survey-Reports/College-Students-Speak_A-Survey-Report-on-Mental-Health-NAMI-2012.pdf

Huta, V. (2015). The complementary roles of eudaimonia and hedonia and how they can be pursued in practice. In S. Joseph (Ed.), *Positive psychology in practice: promoting human flourishing in work, health, education, and everyday life* (2nd ed., pp. 159–182). New York: Wiley. doi:10.1002/9781118996874.ch10

Huta, V. (2016). An overview of hedonic and eudaimonic well-being concepts. In L. Reinecke & M. B. Oliver (Eds.), *Handbook of media use and well-being*. New York: Routledge.

Huta, V., & Ryan, R. M. (2010). Pursuing pleasure or virtue: The differential and overlapping well-being benefits of hedonic and eudaimonic motives. *Journal of Happiness Studies, 11*(6), 735–762. doi:10.1007/s10902-009-9171-4

Huta, V., & Waterman, A. S. (2014). Eudaimonia and its distinction from hedonia: Developing a classification and terminology for understanding conceptual and operational definitions. *Journal of Happiness Studies, 15*(6), 1425–1456. doi:10.1007/s10902-013-9485-0

Jahoda, M. (1958). *Current concepts of positive mental health*. New York: Basic Books. doi:10.1037/11258-000

Keyes, C. L. M. (2002). The mental health continuum: From languishing to flourishing in life. *Journal of Health and Social Behavior, 43*(2), 207–222. doi:10.2307/3090197 PMID:12096700

Keyes, C. L. M. (2010). Mental illness and mental health: The two continua model across the lifespan. *Journal of Adult Development, 17*(2), 110–119. doi:10.1007/s10804-009-9082-y PMID:20502508

Keyes, C. L. M. (2013). Promoting and protecting positive mental health: Early and often throughout the lifespan. In C. L. M. Keyes (Ed.), *Mental well-being: International contributions to the study of positive mental health* (pp. 3–28). Dordrecht: Springer. doi:10.1007/978-94-007-5195-8_1

Keyes, C. L. M., Shmotkin, D., & Ryff, C. D. (2002). Optimizing well-being: The empirical encounter of two traditions. *Journal of Personality and Social Psychology, 82*(6), 1007–1022. doi:10.1037/0022-3514.82.6.1007 PMID:12051575

Levens, S. M., Elrahal, F., & Sagui, S. J. (2016). The role of family support and perceived stress reactivity in predicting depression in college freshman. *Journal of Social and Clinical Psychology*, *35*(4), 342–355. doi:10.1521/jscp.2016.35.4.342

Maher, J. P., Doerksen, S. E., Elavsky, S., Hyde, A. L., Pincus, A. L., Ram, N., & Conroy, D. E. (2012). *A daily analysis of physical activity and satisfaction with life in emerging adults. Health Psychology*. doi:10.1037/a0030129

Malinauskas, B., Raedeke, T., Aeby, V., Smith, J., & Dallas, M. (2006). Dieting practices, weight perceptions, and body composition: A comparison of normal weight, overweight, and obese college females. *Nutrition Journal*, *5*(11), 1475–2891. PMID:16579846

Medline Plus Medical Dictionary. (n. d.). Mental health facts sheet multicultural. Retrieved July 25, 2017, from http://c.merriam-webster.com/medlineplus/Mental%20illness

Milligan, N. V. (2010). Effects of training about academic accommodations on perceptions and intentions of health science faculty. *Journal of Allied Health*, *39*(1), 54–62. PMID:20217008

Morales, E. E. (2014). Learning from success: How original research on academic resilience informs what college faculty can do to increase the retention of low socioeconomic status students. *International Journal of Higher Education*, *3*(3), 92–102. doi:10.5430/ijhe.v3n3p92

National Alliance on Mental Illness. (2012). College students speak: A survey report on mental health. Retrieved March 25, 2017, https://www.nami.org/getattachment/About-NAMI/Publications-Reports/Survey-Reports/College-Students-Speak_A-Survey-Report-on-Mental-Health-NAMI-2012.pdf

National Alliance on Mental Illness. (2014). Mental health facts sheet children and teens. Retrieved March 25, 2017, from https://www.nami.org/getattachment/Learn-More/Mental-Health-by-the-Numbers/childrenmhfacts.pdf

National Alliance on Mental Illness. (2015a). Mental health facts sheet African Americans. Retrieved March 25, 2017, from https://www.nami.org/getattachment/Extranet/NAMI-State-Organization-and-NAMI-Affiliate-Leaders/Awareness/AKA/Mental-Health-Fact-Sheets/AKA-NAMI-African-American-MH-facts.pdf

National Alliance on Mental Illness. (2015b). Mental health facts sheet multicultural. Retrieved March 25, 2017, from http://www.nami.org/NAMI/media/NAMI-Media/Infographics/MulticulturalMHFacts10-23-15.pdf

Pew Research Center. (2011, June 2). Purpose of college education. Retrieved February 9, 2017, from http://www.pewresearch.org/daily-number/purpose-of-college-education/

Ridner, S. L., Newton, K. S., Staten, R. R., Crawford, T. N., & Hall, L. A. (2016). Predictors of well-being among college students. *Journal of American College Health*, *64*(2), 116–124. doi:10.1080/07448481.2015.1085057 PMID:26630580

Rohner, R. P., & Britner, P. A. (2002). Worldwide mental health correlates of parental acceptance-rejection: Review of cross-cultural and intracultural evidence. *Cross-Cultural Research*, *36*(1), 16–47. doi:10.1177/106939710203600102

Ross, L. T., & Hill, E. (2002). Childhood unpredictability, schemas for unpredictability, and risk taking. *Social Behavior and Personality*, *30*(5), 453–473. doi:10.2224/sbp.2002.30.5.453

Ross, L. T., Hood, C. O., & Short, S. (2016). Unpredictability and symptoms of depression and anxiety. *Journal of Social and Clinical Psychology*, *35*(5), 371–385. doi:10.1521/jscp.2016.35.5.371

Ross, L. T., & McDuff, J. (2008). The retrospective family unpredictability scale: Reliability and validity. *Journal of Child and Family Studies*, *17*(1), 13–27. doi:10.1007/s10826-007-9138-1

Ross, L. T., Short, S., & Garofano, M. (2016). Scale of unpredictability beliefs: Reliability and validity. *The Journal of Psychology*, *150*(8), 976–1003. doi:10.1080/00223980.2016.1225660 PMID:27628853

Ryan, R. M., & Deci, E. L. (2001). On happiness and human potentials: A review of research on hedonic and eudaimonic well-being. *Annual Review of Psychology*, *52*(1), 141–166. doi:10.1146/annurev.psych.52.1.141 PMID:11148302

Ryan, R. M., & Deci, E. L. (2001). On happiness and human potentials: A review of research on hedonic and eudaimonic well-being. *Annual Review of Psychology*, *52*(1), 141–166. doi:10.1146/annurev.psych.52.1.141 PMID:11148302

Ryff, C. D. (1989). Happiness is everything, or is it? Explorations on the meaning of psychological well-being. *Journal of Personality and Social Psychology*, *57*(6), 1069–1081. doi:10.1037/0022-3514.57.6.1069

United States Department of Health and Human Services. (n. d.). What Is Mental Health? Retrieved March 18, 2017, from https://www.mentalhealth.gov/basics/what-is-mental-health/

U.S. Department of Education, National Center for Education Statistics. (2012). *The condition of education 2012 (NCES 2012-045), Table A-47-2.*

U.S. Department of Education, National Center for Education Statistics. (2016a). Fast facts: Back to school statistics. Retrieved February 9, 2017, from https://nces.ed.gov/fastfacts/display.asp?id=372

U.S. Department of Education, National Center for Education Statistics. (2016b). *Digest of Education Statistics, 2015 (NCES 2016-014).* Washington, DC: U.S. Department of Education.

U.S. Department of Education, Office of Postsecondary Education. (2015). *Higher Education Act Title II reporting system.* Washington, DC: U.S. Department of Education.

World Health Organization. (2014, August 15). Mental health: A state of well-being. Retrieved February 9, 2017, from http://www.who.int/features/factfiles/menatl_health/en/

Chapter 2
Mental Health and Well-Being:
Societal Influences

Jean Mockry
State University of New York at Plattsburgh, USA

Melissa Martin
State University of New York at Plattsburgh, USA

Alison Puliatte
State University of New York at Plattsburgh, USA

Denise Simard
State University of New York at Plattsburgh, USA

Maureen E. Squires
State University of New York at Plattsburgh, USA

ABSTRACT

In this chapter, the authors provide a brief overview of the distinction between flourishing and non-flourishing mental health and well-being for people not diagnosed with a clinical mental disorder. While recognizing that genetics and personality impact the well-being of people, research supports the profound impact of societal constructs in American life. As part of a team of faculty who work with undergraduate students in Teacher Education, the authors feel this distinction is essential to understand as medical issues require diagnostics by people trained in that area. The book's focus is to examine what the college community can do to promote flourishing mental health in its social construction in classrooms, on campus and beyond. Dominant influences for non-flourishing mental health and well-being for college students rest in ideologies, happiness seeking and digitalization within American life, membership in groups that are underrepresented and well-intentioned but enabling parenting that ill prepares children for adult responses in life.

DOI: 10.4018/978-1-5225-3793-9.ch002

INTRODUCTION

In this chapter, the authors provide a brief overview of the distinction between flourishing and non-flourishing mental health and well-being for people not diagnosed with a clinical mental disorder. While recognizing that genetics and personality impact the well-being of people, research supports the profound impact of societal constructs.

The chapter then focuses on the non-flourishing mental health of undergraduate students in college and the social constructs that have impacted the development of these anxieties. These include the influence of living in American society with its polarizing politics and obsession with the pursuit of happiness and media views of what this looks like, the influence of being a part of groups that are underrepresented in America, such as race and culture, religious beliefs, classism, sexual orientations, gender, and the influence of over-productive parenting and early educational experiences.

NON-FLOURISHING MENTAL HEALTH AND WELL-BEING

No one is raised in a vacuum and this is true of college students. Genetics and environment influence all, and people seeking higher education are no exception. While this life transition can trigger intense feelings of joy, it can also activate feelings of anxiety and depression. For purposes of this book we are not focusing on those with clinical mental illness but rather as Corie Keyes, full professor of Sociology at Emory University and UVM's Keynote for the 2nd Annual Conference "Mental Health Matters: Building a Resilient Campus" (Oct. 28, 2016), identifies those who are struggling emotionally, but who are not classified as mentally ill. He counters the often-held belief that if one does not carry a mental illness then one is mentally healthy, but this denies a category of people who are neither mentally ill nor mentally thriving or flourishing. According to Keyes, this middle category of "not flourishing" can include over 40% of the population.

This chapter will primarily focus on social constructs that can influence mental health and well-being: 1. membership in America's citizenry that promotes the "pursuit of happiness" and the often superficial representation on social media, along with America's current Nationalistic polarization, 2. membership in American's subcommunities that are underrepresented within the larger whole, and 3. membership in families and educational settings that may over-protect and over-control with good intentions, keeping young adults overly dependent on others and insecure in their own abilities and decision making skills. Later in the book there will be information regarding the role the campus community can play in easing some of these social constructs and in building a more supportive, proactive and safe collegiate society.

Using Keyes' Mental Health Continuum, John Fink (2014) identified and analyzed predictors from students about their college experiences that impacted their mental health favorably as college faculty and staff found entering freshmen to have "all-times highs of emotional disengagement" (Fink, 2011, p. 380). The World Health Organization published a report on Promoting Mental Health (2005) that shored the research that mental wellness is more a societal issue that is less about individual interventions and more about "social structures and processes" (p. 29). British author Ruth Whippman in her 2016 book, *America the Anxious: How our pursuit of happiness is creating a nation of nervous wrecks* analyzes America's obsession with happiness and the resulting failure of our intense multiple pursuits of it. She notes that the American Psychological Association (2012), forewarned that the US was on the precipice of "stress-induced public health crisis" (p. 10).

Many would say that it is the larger college community itself, beyond individuals, that creates the climate of stress. A recent study concludes its research with imagining a "different kind of academy, exploring the practices that produce it can be differently enacted…" (Peake, L., & Mullings, B., 2015, p.253). One of the hopes of Peake's and Mullings' study is to begin to create a space for mental wellness that de-stigmatizes people with mental and emotional stress so that care of self is more emphasized and that the corporate mindset of universities is minimized. (273). Whippman recognizes the impact that social media bring to these stresses in chapter 7 entitled, "I'm not a happy person; I just play one on Facebook". The intense need for a positive public persona on social media can result in the creation of a disingenuous self with exaggerated superlative displays of happiness that can play into readers' insecurities as well. This manic polarizing drive to pursue perfect happiness can also result in disconnections from real life and real people.

Informally and in support of the above, we in Teacher Education have observed more students who self-describe themselves as anxious, depressed and overwhelmed in this program so these findings don't surprise us. However, it does challenge us to better understand so we can provide more effective assistance in a systemic and empowering manner, as we acknowledge student responses to frustration, social status and anxiety often run counter to their paths for college success.

THE AMERICAN WAY OF LIFE, PARENTING, AND BRIBERY

The review of literature indicates many influences for non-flourishing mental health on campuses, reflective of the social constructs of communities in which students' live. Beginning in homes with overprotective parenting and/or from parenting immersed in economic survival to students' reactions to the new institutional community they've joined may or may not scaffold this new acclimation. Living in a culture that advocates for 24/7 perfect (and unattainable) happiness presets disappointment for many. People who are from underrepresented groups and who are away from their first home bases may come to realize unique isolation and stressors that might or might not be present for those in the dominant groups. Parenting contributes to mental health status, ironically and particularly from homes that believe they are protecting their children from the world that they believe is difficult to navigate safely (Lythcott-Haims, J., 2015). It's theorized current college students are struggling to find their place in a world with an expansive generation gap, ranging from digital nativism, economic disparities, interpersonal challenges and isolation in spite of life in the world-wide web and a sense of entitlement (Levine, A. & Dean, D., 2012).

At issue for many young college students can be found in Lythcott-Haims' book *How to raise an adult.* She presents a compelling argument that much parenting, while good intentioned, has handicapped young adults who learned to overly rely on protective adults for any decision making, inadvertently undermining their confidence and willingness to take risks, and creating a false expectation that perfection can someway be attained with interventions by authority figures. She argues that current parenting and formal early schooling do a good job of caring for children but a bad job of preparing them to be adults who are independent thinkers and contributors in their adult communities as most of their youths they've been kept safe and involved in adult-decided and supervised recreation and activities. While there are sane reasons for this parenting approach, given milk cartons with many different pictures of children who've been abducted and Halloween candy penetrated with sharp instruments, she thinks this approach went too far and hovering parenting has become the norm. Children have absorbed their parents' fears and tread lightly into the larger world of unknowns. These children have not had enough experiences making their own decisions, such as setting and applying agreed upon rules for pick-up games, where fairness was negotiated among the players. Children have not often had opportunities to recover from incidents dealing with hurt feelings or conflict resolution among themselves. Too often parents become involved to "save" their child from any hurt be it in schools, with peers, with coaches, the list goes on. How do children know they can recover when things don't go the way they'd like? How do they learn to problem solve when there are no problems for them to solve on their own?

Lythcott-Haims says children learn two things from over parenting: they learn they are inept and the world is not safe. This results in passivity, inertia and apprehension. The parent's fears, of which the parent may say is responsibility-taking, turnkeys into insecurity and inaction in the child. An independent, decision making adult has been submerged into a timid, insecure, anxious adult. With good intentions or not.

Jessica Lahey in her book: *The gift of failure: How the best parents learn to let go so their children can succeed* offers a similar sentiment for parents and teachers. She, too, says that over-parenting, of which she concedes complicity from her own parenting, has the potential to undermine children's confidence and undermine their education. Children need many opportunities to have success from their own making or they learn they can't create their successes. Failure is not failure as reputed but rather it is necessary for success to occur. Ms. Lahey learned for herself and now tells others that it is important to embrace children's failures as this is where they learn about life and learn what they can handle on their own.

In this same vein of overprotective parenting, Lukianoff and Hadt perceive colleges campuses and classrooms as over protecting students "from words and ideas students don't like, seeking punishment of those who give even accidental offense" (2015, 42). They build a case showing that guiding students to question their unexamined thinking is challenged with a "new protectiveness" that may encourage pathological thinking and compromised mental health. Reflective of the current culture of polarized politics and hostility and the "self-righteousness fueled by strong partisan emotions" (45), students may feel the pressure to join a side and be true to the "team". The social media used by these true "social-media natives" has shifted the faculty/student balance, putting faculty in fear to offend. Thinking is dominated with strong emotion and defensiveness by both Millennials and Gen Zers, who've received the message from their homes that adults should protect them from the dangers of life, including each other. They further reason, citing psychological theory that people with anxieties need help in facing their fears, not be protected from them.

Many students enter college with the expectations that rewards are attached to everything they do and this could be result of their experiences in K-12 schools and elsewhere. Alfie Kohn espoused the problems with our externally motivated tactics in school operations in his 1993 book, *Punished by rewards: The trouble with gold stars, incentive plans, $, A's, praise and other bribes.* Kohn argues that these "incentives" undermine self-confidence and create a sense that learning is contingent only for the bribe, giving the sense that the learning is secondary. Creative thinking is minimized as getting the bribe becomes the focus and accountability for one's work is greatly diminished as the goal becomes to get through or survive some project, activity, or routine to get to the reward. College students have been well immersed in this world of extrinsic motivation and not enough has been done to develop more fully internal motivation to creatively problem solve and be thoughtfully engaged with the needs of the community in which they live. Rewards become punishments when not received and anxieties can result when the external bribes are not present per expectations.

Daniel Pink in his 2009 book *Drive: The surprising truth about what motivates us* develops this thinking more thoroughly arguing that institutions operate in ways that run counter to science research about what motivates people to engage with full energy in tasks to think deeply and to creatively problem solve. He says the extreme emphasis on rewards and punishment to get work done actually runs counter to learning and problem solving and to the quality of the work. Current young adults have been programmed to do what's minimally expected to get by for a reward or not, but generally not for the joy of the work and/or learning.

Today's college students are living in a world that is very different than their parents, according to Arthur Levine and Diane Dean in *Generation on a tightrope: A portrait of today's college students.* A chart in this book (p. 17, 2012) analyzes four critical areas of difference for today's college students and their parents: technology, globe, economy and demographics. Parents grew up in era where the cold war and two super powered countries thrived. Russia was already dissolved before students were born, and students were babies when the twin towers were attacked by al-Qaeda. They grew up in a world of escalated terrorism and a less powerful nation than the one their parents lived in. Their parents' world was pre-digital (analog) while digital technology is all current students have known. The dominant white middle-aged baby boomer time period in the Northeast and Midwest that parents of current students know has been replaced by many more people from countries other than European heritage, and there's been a shift of living in the NE to the West and South, along with a now aging baby boomer population. Parents' lives began with an economy that was industrial while their children primarily have only known one that is based on information and one that has been in recovery from recession. These social contrasts for students born in the 21st century have been dramatic and realized in a relatively short time period and "give insight into the generational experiences we are experiencing today" (p. 17). In addition, this diverse and different world students inherited "may be far more profound, affecting career choices, economic opportunity and attainment, and the future of the American Dream" (p. 35).

DIVERSITY AND IDENTITY FORMATION

Citing the 1998 study *When Hope and Fear Collide,* Levine and Dean note that the "multicultural divide is less deep; the gap between diverse groups is less wide" (p. 97) and that higher education campuses are not the same as yesteryear. However, they also note that racial, religious and sexual identities are still problematic. And as this digital generation is not strong in interpersonal skills, there is an undercurrent barring good communication and understanding, as does a sense of being political correct. "Diversity problems are one of the topics most frequently left for parents to raise with the dean" (p. 99). Self-segregation by race and lesser by religion is still present on campuses with many students of underrepresented racial and ethnic groups socializing primarily with those in their same groupings. As a result of this inclination there has been a rise in student affinity groups where clubs and organizations are focused on specific populations, such as religious organizations, racial/ethnic and sexual orientation groupings. While these grouping provide assistance to students who are underrepresented in their identity formation, they also can be barrier like to the larger community.

Economic status is a powerful variable in the development of a flourishing mindset. In a December 2015 report from the Pew Research Center entitled. "Parenting in America" it was concluded that there is a notable divide in parenting that is more related to economic circumstances and less for the parenting analysis between the overprotective parenting and the more laid back parental approach for children's life success. Lower income parents have more challenges than higher income families and this shows itself in children's less participation in extracurricular activities, like sports or scouts or the arts and in getting affordable after school care. Social issues like teen pregnancy and legal troubles are higher for those in low SES, and worries about their children being victims of violence are increased too. The heightened propensity for single parenting in the lower SES groups impacts this divide as well. Survivors of those who have lived with poverty have a steeper uphill journey to thrive in colleges.

College students who come from groups that are underrepresented, including students in the LGBTQ community (Sabato, 2016), students who are female (Liss & Erchull, 2015) (Merianos et al., 2013) or students from races that are neither White nor English speaking have different experiences and challenges in college than those in the dominant groups. This "outside looking in" also extends to those students who are from indigenous communities (Scholl, 2006) (Dellinger et al., 2016), to students with different learning abilities (Carroll, Muller & Pattison, 2016) to students who belong to religions other than Christianity (Abdel-Khalek & Lester, 2017). Extra challenges exist for those who are first generation college attenders (Wheeler, 2016), for those in a lower socio-economic status carry (Brown et al., 2015) and/or for those with different abilities (Piers & Duquette, 2016). The campus climate itself may contribute to mental wellness in terms of available supports and sensitivity to the emerging adults' developmental, physical, social, emotional and learning needs.

Identity formation is an integral component of undergraduates' development and a strong indicator of their well-being. Family background, race, ethnicity, religion, sexual orientation, gender and ability can be components of identity as can genetic inclinations and environment that begins with family of birth. It's been found that people with moral and emotional maturity along with identity integration possess more positive mental health and thus engage in fewer risky behaviors (Hardy, 2013). Erik Erikson theorized that there are life stages of psychosocial development, focusing on the crisis for each human in each stage that can conflict with societal expectations. Adolescents search for personal identity in the midst of efforts to clarify their roles in the world to about 18 years of age, the entry age to college. These emerging young adults throughout their undergraduate years in college then search for intimacy as they balance their own sense of isolation. This is where the pursuit of close relationships outside of family develops (McLeod, 2013), and as in all of Erikson's theoretical stages, it is essential for the person to successfully maneuver the elements of "crisis" within each stage and to integrate the skill sets that are necessary for a healthy personality development for life.

This personal life developmental trajectory provides enough hurdles for those born with privileges of belonging to groups in areas such as class, gender, heterosexuality, race, physical, emotional and learning abilities, and language. Even if students' families are familiar with college rigor, demands and expectations, students still need to navigate the new collegiate territory, and this is much more challenging for those without the membership in dominant groups.

For first-generation college students (FGCSs) there may be a lack of grounding in understanding higher education and its operations. In addition, many FGCSs carry the hopes of their families for success and the responsibility to bring them honor and respect. In addition, there may be some intensity around finding careers to support family and this often requires college degrees (Wheeler, 2016). This extra burden can be substantial enough, but if completion of plans or program shifts and the expected success in the career path is at risk, mental wellness may swing toward non-flourishing and as research shows currently, retention of FGCSs is very low compared to other college peers in the first year of college (p. 112). Guilt, a sense of failure and of disappointing family, a belief that the sacrifices of the family make this "failure" difficult to discuss with them in the midst of confusion for next steps can compromise students' mental strength to stay in college and/or approach another career path (p. 114). Compared to their peers, many FGCSs carry a stronger sense of belonging to their families and culture, but when they feel they've broken their commitment to bring honor and improved economic status for their families, this belonging sense can be broken, making them more vulnerable to poorer mental health (p. 115). It's recommended that career counselors understand the uniqueness surrounding the FGCSs' experience in college, so extra steps can be taken to guide and work with them (p. 114).

For students in underrepresented groups of race, culture and/or gender, obstacles for college success and flourishing mental health are present. In a study designed to analyze students from these groups in terms of health wellness compared to White peers, it was found that poorer mental health has a propensity to rest in those from the minority communities, regardless that they may attend colleges where their minority grouping was the majority (Smith, Chesim & Jeglic, 2014). While students who are White may experience social issues around money, academics and entrance into new sub-communities, students who are in the minority also experienced these and additional stressors, such as racism, depression, feelings of isolation, suicidal ideation and self-harm (p. 85). Female students in this study of 461 students ranked at risk for depression, isolation and suicidal ideation as well and if the females were also from the minority racial/ethnic community, there was a higher probability for mental health to not flourish more significantly (85). This study shared a limitation that they didn't distinguish between minorities born in the US and those born elsewhere, so Blacks and Hispanics were situated as one group. It was recommended that this distinction be recognized for a future study (p. 87). There have been many studies from which this study built and it is clear that being from an underrepresented race or culture can impact the well-being of mental health.

Class influences perceptions about higher education. One study used the metaphor of a funnel to better explain "there are "cumulative disadvantage results when first-generation and low-income college students are disproportionately filtered out at each stage of the postsecondary education process: (Aronson, 2007, p. 1). If parents don't possess a college degree, there is a higher likelihood that encouragement for their children to attend college is lessened as ambivalence about dropping out is heightened, as that may reflect their family norm. Financial aid is complex and many students begin in community colleges and try to transfer to 4 year institutions, often with a loss of credits at a financial cost. Academic performance is poorer compared to their more advantaged peers who benefited from a stronger K-12 program.

There is much disparity in readiness for college in terms of what is taught in high schools and college expectations as well as great differences between students living in poverty and those living with economic advantages, parental support and expectations to continue with higher education (Venezia & Jaeger, 2013). Discrepancies are found in schools well-funded from higher SES locations as opposed to those centered in inner cities and rural areas reflecting a lower SES. All public schools are not equal per economic structures that fund public education's resources and programming among low SES public schools, either in urban or rural areas, and this disadvantages students preparing for higher education (Klugman, 2012). The growing stratification within higher education precludes most who are not in the higher SES from attending many selective institutions (p. 803).

As a result, too many students are entering colleges ill prepared for the academic rigor. There's a need for reforms that "take a systemic, comprehensive approach to provide students with both academic (like the CCSS) and nonacademic resources and opportunities" (p. 122) to more comprehensively support students' college readiness needs. Students who are from low SES and those who are first generation to attend college may need to compensate for learning advantages denied them. The additional struggles that students from low SES and those who are first generation impact success at colleges of choice as it influences their mental well-being in juggling feelings of inferiority and feelings of frustration and anxiety in trying to keep up with the college work and often with employment to augment college costs.

Keyes, et al (2010) concluded that genetics play a role in influencing social and emotional health, as does environment. Burris, et al analyzed several factors that contributed to students' psychological distress and well-being. Among them they found that the best predictor of positive mental health was a positive disposition (2009). Students who can see the glass half full rather than half empty demonstrate perseverance in their studies and work. This study also found that students who see their health as important (HAV-Health as value) also have better mental health. Exercise, good nutrition and minimizing alcohol intake show a positive indicator for better mental health. More study is needed to connect religiousness, spirituality and sexual behaviors but there are indicators these, too, could be predictors.

Supporting Keyes' research, Fink explored elements that could predict student mental health in college life (2014). Keyes had developed a mental health continuum, describing positive social functioning and the implicit optimism in working with and expectations of individuals and groups to be indicators of mental health from languishing to flourishing. Fink added Astin's I-E-O conceptual framework that identifies input, environment and outcome to project how precollege characteristics along with the college's environments could reflect scores that indicate flourishing mental health. While this study highlighted several predictors of flourishing mental health for college students, such as supportive social arenas, ease into college routine, sense of belonging and self-confidence, this study didn't show relationship with students' college environs and positive mental health.

Levine and Dean have also found that there are differences in thinking and attitude in this generation of Blacks, Whites, Hispanics, Asian Americans, Females and Males in being less polarized with race and gender and having more satisfaction with college. They've expressed a community feeling, having professors who are accessible, experiencing good teaching quality and having comfort with expressing unpopular or controversial positions. There is more positivity regarding race and discrimination and opportunities for women than in their parents' generation. "There is more homogeneity between groups and greater heterogeneity within diverse groups than in the past as well" (p. 107).

However, as social constructs are considered in analyzing non-flourishing mental health for college students, there needs to be mention of the dramatic shift in US leadership this year of 2017. "A culture of war buttressed by the forces of white supremacy and militarization has been unleashed in a series of policies designed to return the United States to a history in which the public sphere was largely white and Christian, and the economy was and the state were governed by a ruling corporate elite" (Giroux 2017, p. 1). We are experiencing a pugilistic attitude at home with Muslims, women and their reproductive rights, immigrants and the poor, along with the sense that war abroad could happen at a tweet's moment. Giroux argues that those with social liberal perspectives need to pay attention to the politics and the causations for this shift in leader shift, this polarization of citizens who are passionate about being ignored, losing good jobs and benefits and who are looking to a hero to save them. Emotions are high and fear is widespread from both polarized positions of those believing the current POTUS can right the ship to those fearful of his capricious, erratic functioning.

Just prior to his election in fall 2016, some of these fears were articulated in a journal that re-constructed his Nationalistic slogan, "Make America great again" to "Make America hate again". Rage was and is widespread in reaction to a slowed economy, terrorism, social and demographic transitions, mass shootings, crime and gun control, in addition to leadership that well knows how to manipulate these emotions for personal benefits. Sasha Abramsky describes hateful behaviors toward Islam, Muslims, immigrants and those not white. She says this "rejection of democratic norms" will be felt for years to come not only in the US but around the world (Abramsky 2016, p. 29). As a land of immigrants and people of diversity in religion, culture, race, language and sexual orientations, those in these groups, at college or not, may have a higher propensity toward non-flourishing mental health and those of us in public and private institutions need to shore each other with support and strategies for coping with this public state of affairs. Polarization in thinking has threatened engaging conversations to understand and compromise with the other.

One study about traits of college students identified several factors that contribute to what the researcher called "the mental health crisis in North America". Based in Canada but inclusive of the United States' populations, Kruisselbrink Flatt (2013) cites a study that determined that depression in Canadian and US institutions found first year students met the criteria for depression with 7% being male and 14% being female. She notes that nearly 100% of campus psychological counseling centers have reported a rise of cases with students seeking mental health interventions. In this paper, she notes several factors that contribute to this "crisis", with academic pressure being first with the high-grade expectations, the reality check for this and millennials difficulty in dealing with failure. The competitive economic environment also creates strain for employment probabilities, along with student loan debt increasing the more years in higher education to prepare for life after. Kruisselbrink found in her research that it wasn't the amount of the debt that was the stressor but rather it was the students' worry about the debt that impacted their academic performance in a negative manner. Another factor cited was the accessibility of higher education for those from lower SES brackets who previously wouldn't have had this option to further their education, speculating that the competitive college environment may trigger for some college students from disadvantaged backgrounds mental health stressors as survivors of less than desirable home environments.

In a March 2014 study, the Pew Research Center focused on "Millennials in Adulthood" and found that "they are relatively unattached to organized politics and religion, linked by social media, burdened by debt, distrustful of people, in no rush to marry and optimistic about the future" (p. 1). They also describe them as "America's most racially diverse generation" (p. 2). In spite of their optimism, they also carry more debt than the previous generations of Gen Xers and Boomers as a result of the convergence of The Great Recession, globalization and rapid technological change on the American workforce. Millennials that are only equipped with a high school degree particularly feel this divide with higher unemployment and lower wages than those in previous generations. It is not a stretch to understand Millennials lack of trust of institutions and their critiquing of those in charge, such as politicians, priests/ministers/rabbis etc. teachers/professors, management personnel and decision makers. According to this report, that while Millennials vote Democratic, more than half choose "not to identify with either political party" (p. 8).

Levine and Dean find that Millennials are very conflicted. They are passionate about desiring social change as Obama promised but find themselves disillusioned with social institutions and they have disengaged from social activism with outspoken liberal leaning but conservative beliefs and the conservative identification but liberal positions. It's as if they refuse to fit in any mold (p. 131). The environment and globe tend to bring them together as a group. They overwhelmingly say they want to make a difference in the world, and it appears global environmental issues and local issues tend to be more on their radars. However, "Their commitment is not large-a median and mode of eleven to twenty hours a year" (p. 146).

Levine and Dean discuss the irony of technology usage for Millennials and Gen Zers that brings social life into the classroom while replacing the need for social life on campus. They discuss the "new tribalism" in which social media contacts can expand to present and past friends, family and any number of people 24/7 in class and out, creating their virtual communities and a lack of need for face to face relationships. The existence of diaphobe which is "the fear of being without a digital device" (p. 75), creates an inherent intense focus on the device in which some would say much time is wasted. With this comes the expectation that everyone else is reading texts and email as soon as they are sent and that the expectation for an instant response creates impatience and a sense that Millennials and Gen Zers are the "I want it now generation" (p. 75). We know fellow college instructors who share both frustration and feelings of anxiety around the emails late at night to answer questions re: coursework. Synchronous time overlaps with students with asynchronous time. Many faculty want to help students as much as possible, but maybe not at midnight. Many students expect answers when they ask the questions. And many students obfuscate social media "friends' with genuine ones. The social navigation remains complicated in spite of technological advances.

An Undergraduate Survey 2009 shows that more than a third of undergraduates do not participate in the general social activities on campus like: the gym or fitness center, academic or professional clubs, lectures, debates, or other academic events. The library is one exception. Part of this finding is that more students need to "work longer hours, attend college part time, and extend undergraduate education beyond age twenty-four" (p.57) in at least State schools and community colleges. However, this is not the only causation for less involvement in campus activities. In three studies in response to the question about what they like to do for fun, drinking and partying were number one response. This isn't a new phenomenon but how and what they drink may be. They are not drinking beer in the same way but rather they drink hard alcohol with flavored vodka as a new favorite. They also drink more intensely, not just five or six but often twelve or more (p. 60). And as a result, as always when alcohol is in the mix, good decision making is compromised. Sexual encounters, harassment, stalking, violence, drug use other than alcohol can be advanced and the next day's regret can contribute to non-flourishing mental health.

Boundaries have been blurred for Millennials and Gen Zers as a result of public posting and the needed self-restraint to think before response posting. As a result, stalking has escalated and this is not easy to differentiate from checking out others' posts which might be called voyeuristic but not with carried intent to invade another's space for harm. From the 2009 Undergraduate Survey quoted by Levine and Dean, nearly half of the undergraduates "believe they can trust the people they meet through Facebook" (p. 76). Strong emotions result when they find this isn't always true.

While today's college students are not the people of yesteryear, this has been said of young people by older people for decades, if not centuries. We do, however, have a better profile of who we are teaching when we consider the research. We know we have many more people in our classrooms that come from underrepresented groups; we have people who have always lived with full immersion into technological access; we have people who may need to shore their interpersonal skills, who are more comfortable online communicating than they are in person; we have people who have lived in economic times that are less secure financially than their parents were with less hope to improve their quality of living as had been the expectation of earlier generations; simultaneously, we have people who are more impulsive consumers who want what they want when they want it; we have people who have been over protected and not given enough opportunities to think and act on their own accord and as a result expect life to go their way with minimal effort, on their part.

We also have college students who are more comfortable with diversity than previous generations. They are experienced technologically savvy, networking as they think globally rather than "in a flattened world" (p. 163). They have potential to become genuine multiculturally competent humans with needed digital expertise in this global society.

Our future work on campus centers around the question: How do we help undergraduates manage their anxieties for more flourishing mental health and well-being, so they can access their talents for their own personal developments and that of the communities in which they live? Much of their non-flourishing selves finds causation within the communities in which they have lived. We as faculty are building our own mindfulness as we move forward to address strategies to help our students manage their lives for their own well-being. The following chapters will speak to character trait development, emotional intelligence awareness and campus-wide initiatives, in addition to our thinking about "next steps". We know there is no perfect as we also believe we can do better tomorrow.

REFERENCES

Aronson, P. (2008). Breaking barriers or locked out? Class-based perceptions and experiences of postsecondary education. *New Directions for Child and Adolescent Development*, *2008*(119), 41–54. doi:10.1002/cd.208 PMID:18330921

Fink, J. (2014). Flourishing: Exploring Predictors of Mental Health Within the College Environment. *Journal of American College Health, 62*(6), 380–388. doi:10.1080/07448481.2014.917647 PMID:24779485

Giroux, H. A. (2017). White nationalism, armed culture and state violence in the age of Donald Trump. *Philosophy & Social Critics.* doi:10.1177/0191453717702800

Keyes, C., Kendler, K., Myers, J., & Martin, C. (2014). The Genetic Overlap and Distinctiveness of Flourishing and the Big Five Personality Traits. *Journal of Happiness Studies, 16*(3), 655–668. doi:10.1007/s10902-014-9527-2

Klugman, J. (2012). How Resource Inequalities Among High Schools Reproduce Class Advantages in College Destinations. *Research in Higher Education, 53*(8), 803–830. doi:10.1007/s11162-012-9261-8

Kohn, A. (1993). *Punished by rewards: The trouble with gold stars, incentive plans$, A's, Praise, and other bribes.* Boston: Houghton Mifflin.

Kruisselbrink Flatt, A. (2013). A Suffering Generation: Six Factors Contributing to the Mental Health Crisis in North American Higher Education. *College Quarterly, 16*(1).

Levine, A., & Dean, D. (2012). *Generation on a tightrope: A portrait of today's college student.* San Francisco: Jossey-Bass.

Lythcott-Haims, *J.* (2015). *Summary and analysis of How to raise an adult: Break free of the over parenting trap and prepare your children for success.* New York: St. Martin's Press.

Peake, L., & Mullings, B. (2015). Critical Reflection on Mental and Emotional Distress in the Academy. Toronto, Ontario; Queens University.

Pew Research Center. (2014. March 14). Millennials in adulthood: Detached from Institutions, networked with friends. Retrieved from www.pewsocialtrends.org/2014/03/07/millennialsinadulthood/

Pew Research Center. (2015, December 17). *Parenting in America: Outlook, worries, aspirations are strongly linked to financial situation.* Retrieved from www.pewsocialtrends.org/2015/12/17/parenting-in-america/

Pink, D. (2009). *Drive: The surprising truth about what motivates us.* San Francisco: Josse-Bass.

Smith, K., Chesin, M., & Jeglic, E. (2014). Minority College Student Mental Health: Does Majority Status Matter? Implications for College Counseling Services. *Journal of Multicultural Counseling and Development*, *42*(2), 77–92. doi:10.1002/j.2161-1912.2014.00046.x

Whippman, R. (2016). *America, the Anxious: How our pursuit of happiness is making us nervous wrecks.* New York: St. Martin's Press.

Chapter 3
Dispositional Factors Influencing College Success:
Personality, Character, and Mindset

Melissa Martin
State University of New York at Plattsburgh, USA

Jean Mockry
State University of New York at Plattsburgh, USA

Alison Puliatte
State University of New York at Plattsburgh, USA

Denise Simard
State University of New York at Plattsburgh, USA

Maureen E. Squires
State University of New York at Plattsburgh, USA

ABSTRACT

Attending college can be difficult for some students. Fong and Loi (2015) noted that these challenges may be the result of attending school in a different city/town away from home, missing family or friends, or balancing the requirements of school with work. Because of this, some students "experience substantial distress" while in school (Fong & Loi, 2015). So, why do students handle stress differently? Perhaps personality, character dispositions, and mindsets impact a student's ability to manage stress. More specifically, a student's grit, self-control, resilience, and self-compassion may impact the student's ability to handle challenges while in college. The authors also discuss how these character dispositions impact a specific audience – preservice general and special educators enrolled in coursework to become K-12 teachers.

DOI: 10.4018/978-1-5225-3793-9.ch003

INTRODUCTION

College can be challenging for some students for various reasons including being away from home and balancing the demands of work and school (Fong & Loi, 2015). Because of this, some students "experience substantial distress" while in school (Fong & Loi, 2015). Distress may include negative emotions, stress, depression, or burnout (Fong & Loi, 2015). An abundance of stress from these challenges can impact your *well-being* (Neely, Schallert, Mohammed, Roberts, & Chen, 2009), which is described as how you function (Fong & Loi, 2015).

There are two types of well-being: (1) hedonic, and (2) eudaimonic (Fong & Loi, 2015). The first type is also often referred to as *subjective well-being*. Zessin, Dickhauser, and Garbade (2015) described this type as "how people evaluate their life, including emotional and cognitive judgments" (p. 341). Cognitive evaluation refers to your satisfaction with your life, while the emotional judgements evaluate pleasant versus negative affect (Zessin, Dickhauser, & Garbade, 2015).

The second type of well-being is eudaimonic, which is referred to as *psychological well-being*. That is, the ability to personally grow and have self-acceptance (Fong & Loi, 2015). This is the type of well-being you often read about in literature – it often refers to *flourishing* or *non-flourishing* well-being. According to researchers, this type is the "pursuit of realization of one's true potential and focuses on the optimal functioning of the individual" (p. 341; Zessin, et al., 2015).

Although much of the research related to well-being describes subjective and psychological, Zessin and colleagues (2015) also noted other types. They posited that happiness, your relationships with others, and your spiritual beliefs impact your ability to function. To the lay person, this makes sense. If we have conflict with a friend or partner, we may have a negative affect, which can ultimately impact other parts of our life (e.g., work or school). We may not be as focused (or are distracted) and have difficulty managing or balancing all parts of our life. This may, also, impact our happiness. If there is a chronic conflict, we may become unhappy, which, again, can lead to negative results in other areas of our lives.

As Fong and Loi (2015) noted, college can be challenging for students. But, let's face it - we all have stress. Perhaps our stress is not continuous (or chronic), but rather situational (or acute). Additionally, we do not all have the same background factors (as described in the previous chapter) that may exacerbate our stress levels. Either way, we all handle stressors differently. Some *seem* to handle stress effortlessly, while others seem to handle it poorly. We all know the people who shut down when life becomes too overwhelming, and we also know the people who fight stress head on. So, why do our reactions differ?

The type of stress may influence our reaction. If a negative event occurs in our life that we believe we can solve, we may feel less stress. But, we may have elevated stress levels for events we do not believe can be easily solved. For example, perhaps we are feeling stress because a large paper is due in a couple of days. But, we have confidence we can write effectively and are prepared to complete this task. On the other hand, what if our car dies because of the frigid temperatures? We may not be as confident in fixing cars, or, perhaps, we are in a financial strain which may impact our ability to get it fixed professionally. Would one situation have a higher level of stress?

For some, however, any type of stressor may cause a reaction, regardless of the situation or type. So, why do some of us seem to handle stress more effectively than others? What makes some people better "adjusters" than others? Throughout this chapter, we will explore some of options as to why some people may handle stress differently. First, we explore why discussing stress is important for a specific audience – preservice general and special educators.

STRESS AND TEACHERS

For this chapter, we focus on how stress can impact college students enrolled in teacher preparation programs. Specifically, we focus on how character dispositions of students who are preservice general and special educators can impact them in college. Additionally, and perhaps more importantly, we also discuss why these dispositions will be important once these students become teachers in public and private K-12 schools.

First, it is important to note that teachers have stress. In fact, The *MetLife Survey of the American Teacher: Challenges for School Leadership*, which was published in 2012, explored teacher satisfaction and challenges related to the teaching profession (MetLife Inc., 2013). The researchers surveyed 1,000 teachers and 500 principals across the United States. Results indicated that more than half of teachers (51%) deal with "great stress several days a week"

(MetLife Inc., 2013). Moreover, the Gallup-Healthways Well-Being Index was administered to over 9,000 teachers in 2013 (Lopez & Sidhu, 2013). This Index examined the well-being of respondents. Results indicated teachers rank their lives higher than almost all other jobs (Index = 68.8). However, almost half (47%) of respondents indicated they have "high levels of stress" daily. In fact, teachers ranked the second highest in this category when examining the relation between occupation and stress (Lopez & Sidhu, 2013).

Therefore, teachers are often faced with daily stressors. They must interact with a variety of people – including students, parents, administrators, and other faculty members. They must also plan instruction based on a variety of needs from all diverse learners in their classrooms. So, it is essential preservice teachers have the tools to handle these stressors before they become full time teachers in K-12 classrooms. It is also important to have the needed character dispositions to be able to cope with these stressors. These may include grit, self-control, resilience, and self-compassion. We discuss these dispositions in this chapter and how they can impact a student in college and teachers in the field. But first, we briefly address another possible reason why some people may handle stress differently – our personalities.

PERSONALITY TRAITS

Researchers are beginning to examine the relationship between well-being and personality traits (Keyes, Kendler, Myers, & Martin, 2015). These traits are defined as "descriptions of people in terms of relatively stable patterns of behavior, thoughts, and emotions" (p. 3; Parks-Leduc, Feldman, & Bardi, 2015). Researchers often use the Big Five personality model to describe such descriptions (Komarraju, Karua, & Schmeck, 2009). This model identifies five personality characteristics including conscientiousness, openness, neuroticism, extraversion, and agreeableness (Anglim & Grant, 2016). Although, we realize personality may impact college success and, certainly, your well-being while in school, the purpose of this chapter is to explore other factors including character dispositions (i.e., non-cognitive skills) and mindsets (fixed and growth).

CHARACTER DISPOSITIONS

One reason for various reactions to distress may be caused by different character dispositions. That is, the traits we inherit or grow. These traits (positive or negative) may impact our well-being. We will discuss four traits throughout this chapter that may impact our mental health, thus our ability to function in college.

Grit

Research indicates, perhaps, a college student who has grit can handle stressors more effectively than other students, and rise to the challenges of college and other stressors (Vainino & Daukantaite, 2015). *Grit*, which is defined as having both a passion and the ability to persevere, may be attributed to less negative effects of distress (Duckworth, 2016; Duckworth, Quinn, & Seligman, 2009). A key of grit is that it is withstanding, meaning grit is not short term. Rather, it refers to long term goals (Duckworth et al., 2009). Because of this, grittier students are often more successful than those who do not have long-term commitment. Perhaps, students who are passionate are more likely to persevere through challenges. These students are often more successful than those who (a) are less gritty, and (b) are academically superior. That is, students who are intelligent and with-it academically may not be more successful than those who identify as gritty. Vainino and Daukantaite (2015) noted that "[g]rit has been shown to predict success over and above the effects of IQ…" (p. 2120).

This is an important note. According to research, you could be academically inferior and still be successful. For example, a student could aim to become a special education teacher. This student, perhaps, is passionate about helping students with special needs and is "all-in," meaning that this student will not only be engaged in coursework as well as complete assignments eagerly and effectively, but will also seek to learn as much information as possible about special education. This passion will promote perseverance when faced with challenges. For example, let's say this student has several assignments due at midterm for her special education coursework in college. The passion (in this case, desire to learn as much as possible about this topic) will ultimately promote effort. This student, instead of becoming overwhelmed and giving up or submitting subpar work, will persevere and put in the work to accomplish his/her tasks (and thus his/her long-term goals). On the flip side, if a less gritty student, who is taking the same coursework as the above described scenario, is feeling stressed about midterms, s/he may not put in the effort to accomplish the tasks if s/he is not passionate about special education. Even if this student has a high IQ, s/he may not persevere through the challenges of this time of the semester and be "all-in." Thus, the student who lacks grit may actually not perform as well as the student who is not as intelligent.

Duckworth (2016) described a similar situation. She examined the cadets who attended the Military Academy at West Point, which is a prestigious honor if accepted into this rigorous program. Research indicates the cadets who were gritty fared better than those who were not. Grit was a more important factor than other scores (e.g., SAT, ACT). In other words, those at the tops of their classes were not always the most successful; those who were grittier were.

So, why are gritty students often more successful than those with high intelligence who are not gritty? This is likely because the definition of grit encompasses two important characteristics, or traits, of these students: passion and perseverance. Muenks and colleagues (2016) noted that passion involves having a "consistency of interests." This makes sense because grit is long-term. In other words, a fleeting passion may not make you gritty. For example, at New Year's you may have a passion for exercising. Perhaps you have promised to begin consistently exercising as part of a resolution for the year. Although you may be interested at the moment, if exercising is not a passion of yours, you are probably not gritty in this area of your life. This fleeting passion may not last and could be situational (resolution) instead of a long-term commitment. Because of this, grit may not help you persevere to put in the effort to consistently exercise and to keep this resolution.

Thus, grit differs from the Big Five personality trait of conscientiousness (Muenks, et al., 2016). Conscientiousness, although related to grit, can be short term (or fleeting). Unlike grit, a student can possess this personality trait for short periods of time (Muenks, et al., 2016). We can use this example with our exercise scenario. We may possess conscientiousness to exercise regularly to lose weight, but this may not be a lasting interest. Thus, in the short term, it may help us achieve our goal, but this commitment may not last. Perhaps, after we lose the targeted amount of weight, we quit exercising because it was just a momentary (short term) goal and not a lasting passion.

Additionally, Vainio and Daukantaite (2015) posited that grit is malleable and can be changed through intervention or support. As educators, we, perhaps, can help our students in college become gritty. The key may be to help students find their passions. A student who is not majoring in a subject of deep interest may lose focus when faced with challenges. If a student does not want to major in an area of passion, perhaps extracurricular activities (e.g., art, dance, music, athletics) will provide purpose and help that student find their gritty-selves.

In education, we want gritty teachers to work with diverse students including those with different abilities. Teachers who are not "all in" and do not put in the effort to succeed may quickly give up when faced with challenges. For example, a teacher may have several students with special needs (e.g., learning disabilities, Autism Spectrum Disorder). If educating students is not a passion, this educator may not be willing to put in the effort to learn how to reach (and teach) these students. This may mean some of the students have failing grades because of ineffective teaching and/or a lack of rapport with the students (because they realize this teacher does not care enough to grow)– neither are qualities of an effective educator.

We may need to try to grow grit in those who do not already possess this characteristic. Because this trait is malleable, we can plan supports in the college classroom to help students develop passion and perseverance. We will discuss how to promote grit and other character traits in the next chapter.

Self-Control

Self-control is another beneficial characteristic to possess when dealing with the stressors of college life. Tangney and colleagues (2004) defined this construct as the "capacity to change and adapt the self so as to produce better, more optimal fit between self and world" (p. 275). A major component of this trait is composure. That is, those who have self-control can refrain from reacting (either good or bad) immediately. This may impact the way we speak to others and our habits.

Have you ever said something to a friend or colleague that you regret? Perhaps, in this instance, you should have refrained from reacting (in this case, speaking) before collecting your thoughts. Instead, you had a knee-jerk reaction in which you responded without a calming filter. People with self-control can "refrain from acting" out (Tangney, Baumeister, & Boone, 2004) and do not succumb to impulsivity (Park, Wright, Pais, & Ray, 2016). Instead, they gain their composure before responding. This may lead to being more effective communicators (and let's face it, less regrets).

In college, students are often faced with many temptations. There are often parties every night, new friends to make, and, sometimes, alcohol and drugs. These can all be tempting to young adults. Students who lack self-control may not be able to stop going out when they should be studying or completing coursework. Rather, they go out with friends several nights per week, which may negatively impact their time commitment to their coursework. Conversely, some students may obsess over studying and coursework. They lack self-control to know when enough is enough. This may lead to burnout from overexertion.

Moreover, students who lack self-control may have difficulty saying "no" to others. For example, an employer may ask the student to work overtime to fill in for another employee who failed to show up for work. Students with "self-control depletion" (Park et al., 2016) may not make the best choice in terms of academics. Perhaps this student has an exam or two the next day and needs to study. Instead, s/he decided to work overtime, thus reducing the time allowed for coursework. This could negatively impact sleep and grades.

Perhaps stress initiates some bad habits (e.g., overeating). These students may eat (or drink, etc.) to feel better when in distress. Students with "self-control depletion" may not be able to stop these habits, leading to negative effects or consequences. Self-control could help prevent negative habits and promote positive well-being.

In the college classroom, students may need to use self-control when communicating with others. Perhaps, during a lecture, students may not agree with the instructor's (or classmate's) perspective. Being able to communicate a differing point of view takes tack and self-awareness. If a student lacks self-control, s/he may not take the time to speak effectively. Rather, s/he may blurt out impulsively. This can negatively impact the classroom environment.

Additionally, in college, students are often required to work cooperatively on assignments. Self-control is an important characteristic during this time, as well. Students will need to contribute equal amounts of work and communicate effectively to work together.

In college, instructors may need to help students gain perspective and self-control because this is an important trait for teachers to possess. There are many challenging situations that will occur in which a teacher may want to act impulsively (e.g., dealing with parents and administrators). A parent may be frustrated and unhappy with your performance. A teacher will have to possess self-control to refrain from reacting without a filter. Instead of becoming defensive and communicating impulsively, teachers with high self-control will choose words carefully and respond professionally first.

Resilience

Another important trait of successful college students (and later as teachers) is resilience. This construct is defined as the ability to adapt to challenges (Hartley, 2011; Fergus & Zimmerman, 2005). Hartley (2011) noted that college life may be stressful to approximately a third of students. Therefore, if you have a college class of 30 students, about 10 of those students are likely experiencing hardships or challenges during the time in your class.

Resilience is the way in which a student overcomes these challenges. Perhaps, a college student received a poor grade on an assignment that required a lot of effort. Students lacking the fortitude to "move on" may dwell on the negative grade. Perhaps these students may lose motivation to continue the course, or quit attending class. Those with resilience, however, may devise a plan to do better in the future - perhaps study more effectively or devote more time to the assignment. Hartley (2011) attributed resilience to "explain why some individuals behave adaptively under great stress" (p. 596). These students can "bounce back" easily and cope with challenges (Tugade & Fredickson, 2004).

Additionally, in teacher education, a student may need the trait of resilience to cope with a negative teaching evaluation. Perhaps the evaluator noted areas of concern or areas of needed improvement when observing the preservice teacher with children. Preservice teachers who are resilient will not dwell on the negativity (perhaps consider dropping out of the program because they perseverate on the negative and deem themselves unfit to teach). Instead, they will bounce back and use that information in the future.

As noted, college students experience a plethora of hardships outside of the classroom, too. The ability to adapt and cope is crucial. For example, a college student could also be dealing with stressors from back home. Perhaps, a relative is gravely sick and the student must deal with that reality while attending school (and possibly working). Resilience is needed to not give in and lose hope. Coping strategies may need to be implemented in the college classroom to promote these skills.

Although we (as college educators) believe students need training in the area of resilience, it is important to note that resilience may be misperceived by students. A student could believe s/he is resilient, yet, in actuality, not be at all. Hartley (2011) conducted a study with about 600 college students and found a disconnect between the students who identified themselves as being able to tolerate stress and their grade point average (GPA). That is, some students indicated they had high stress tolerance, yet had low GPAs. Therefore, as with many constructs, perception is everything. Instructors could implement interventions and strategies in the college classrooms to an audience believing they possess this trait (among others). This may mean we need to also provide examples and non-examples of resilient behavior to awaken some self-awareness in these young adults.

Being a resilient teacher is also important. Not every school day will be good. The children will test boundaries, the lesson plans will fail, and the paperwork will stack up. But, resilient teachers will overcome these obstacles and be the best teachers they can be for their students. They will not get too discouraged. Instead, they will adapt and use their experiences (good or bad) to improve and move forward.

Self-Compassion

Finally, *self-compassion* may impact how we treat ourselves. This character trait is defined as having compassion towards ourselves (i.e., self-kindness). Specifically, Neff and colleagues (2010) described this trait as referring "to the ability to hold one's feelings of suffering with a sense of warmth, connection, and concern" (p. 226). Fong and Loi (2015) noted that we may have compassion for others during challenging times, but we often lack that trait when evaluating our own difficulties. Instead of viewing our stress (or mistakes) critically, those with this trait approach their struggles with compassion.

Self-compassion has three components including (1) self-kindness, (2) common humanity, and (3) mindfulness. Students ascribing to self-kindness believe they deserve love, no matter the magnitude of their mistakes (Barnard & Curry, 2011). These students approach difficulties with forgiveness and love instead of judging themselves critically (Barnard & Curry, 2011). Common humanity refers to our desire to connect (opposite of isolation) and accept that sometimes we are imperfectly human. Finally, mindfulness is accepting the present "as is" and not reacting (Barnard & Curry, 2011; Hall, Row, Wuensch, & Godley, 2013). The common theme of this trait is acceptance and forgiveness.

This trait is important for college students. Those who, perhaps, perform poorly in a course may harbor resentment towards themselves or be overly critical. These students may have difficulty moving past this experience. They may harbor these feelings and find it challenging to forgive themselves. Some of these students may self-identify as perfectionists. They expect perfection-no matter the task. These students may find it difficult to accept imperfections as a part of life. Students who are self-compassionate, however, accept the grade (remember, they are mindful) and do not over-think or over-analyze the situation. These students can move forward and forgive themselves.

This may be especially important if a student, perhaps, did not put forth the effort needed to complete an assignment effectively. Perhaps, this student made a poor choice (lack of self-control, maybe) and did not exert the effort s/he knew was needed. The result was a bad grade. Students who lack the trait of self-compassion may find it very challenging to move on. Perhaps, they over-compensate and are very hard on themselves. Kindness and forgiveness would likely be needed in this situation.

Fong and Loi (2015) noted that self-compassion is related to well-being. Therefore, the students who can forgive themselves are likely to function better and have less distress. These students do not stress over the grade or assignment. Instead, they can compartmentalize and be kind to themselves.

As a teacher, we constantly rely on self-compassion, too. Some lessons will flop – no matter how creative or how much thought you put into it. Sometimes the chips do not fall your way. It is essential to not hold grudges with yourself. Learn from it and move on. Constantly harboring on the poor lesson may also cause burnout or unhappiness, which can ultimately impact our well-being.

MINDSETS

Another variable to a student's well-being may be his/her *mindset*, which is the way in which we view intelligence and our other capabilities. Dweck and Leggett (1988) identified two different types of mindsets: performance goal oriented versus mastery goal oriented. This view of themselves may impact effort and could, potentially, impact how they handle challenges.

Students who are performance goal oriented exert effort to receive praise from others and believe their intelligence is fixed. In other words, no matter how hard they work, they cannot get smarter. Students with this entity view of intelligence believe their competence is out of their control (uncontrollable) – no matter how much effort is exerted (Dweck & Leggett, 1988). This is a fixed mindset.

Conversely, students who are mastery goal oriented believe their intelligence is malleable; that is, it can be changed. Students with this incremental view of intelligence believe they can work hard (i.e., exert effort) and become smarter or more competent. Additionally, students who subscribe to this mindset are not afraid to tackle challenges because, according to this theory, they are ultimately in control of their success. This is a growth mindset (Dweck & Leggett, 1988).

These two very different mindsets may impact college students in and out of the classroom. Students with a fixed mindset may give up quickly because they do not see a path in which they will be successful. For example, a student may receive a poor grade on an exam or project. Instead of taking ownership of that grade (and even brainstorming reasons why they received that grade), these students believe they did all they could and, perhaps, even attribute this grade to other reasons other than themselves (e.g., teacher bias). Students with a growth mindset, however, view this grade as an opportunity to grow and learn more. They use this failure as a spark to grow as a student and learner.

Outside of school, these mindsets can have an impact, too. When faced with the opportunity to go out with friends or stay home and study, students with a fixed mindset may decide there is no reason to study (which could also be attributed to self-control depletion). Instead of electing to exert the effort needed to do well in school, these students may decide no amount of effort will be good enough. Students with growth mindsets, however, seem to embrace challenges and may make a different decision regarding going out or staying in to study.

As educators, we want our preservice general and special educators to believe intelligence is malleable and put forth the needed effort to improve. As we have indicated throughout this chapter, teaching is challenging and filled with stressors. Teachers need to be willing to grow to become the best educators who meet the needs of diverse groups of students. A growth mindset may be key to promoting the effort needed to become effective educators.

CONCLUSION

The complex nature and interconnectedness of personality, character, and mindset can make college life tricky. This chapter described three possible reasons some people seem to handle stress differently, but it is not always that simplistic. For example, we could view intelligence as malleable (growth mindset) but lack self-control, grit, or other character dispositions that help us make good choices in school. Regardless of the reason why we handle stress differently, it is important students have coping strategies they can employ when faced with stressors. Importantly, preservice teachers need tools to take with them after graduation when they become K-12 teachers in the field. Because teachers are often faced with stressors (Lopez & Sidhu, 2013; MetLife, 2013), it may be essential for college educators to help them learn how to cope. The next chapter will explore some strategies to incorporate mindfulness and other tools to help college students handle stress.

REFERENCES

Anglim, J., & Grant, S. (2016). Predicting psychological and subjective well-being from personality: Incremental prediction from 30 facts over the big 5. *Journal of Happiness Studies*, *17*(1), 59–80. doi:10.1007/s10902-014-9583-7

Barnard, L. K., & Curry, J. F. (2011). Self-compassion: Conceptualizations, correlates, and interventions. *Review of General Psychology*, *15*(4), 289–303. doi:10.1037/a0025754

Duckworth, A. (2016). *Grit: The power of passion and perseverance*. New York, NY: Scribner.

Duckworth, A. L., Quinn, P. D., & Seligman, M. E. P. (2009). Positive predictors of teacher effectiveness. *The Journal of Positive Psychology*, *4*(6), 540–547. doi:10.1080/17439760903157232

Dweck, C. S., & Leggett, E. L. (1988). A social-cognitive approach to motivation and personality. *Psychological Review*, *95*(2), 256–273. doi:10.1037/0033-295X.95.2.256

Fergus, S., & Zimmerman, M. A. (2005). Adolescent resilience: A framework for understanding healthy development in the face of risk. *Annual Review of Public Health*, *26*(1), 399–419. doi:10.1146/annurev.publhealth.26.021304.144357 PMID:15760295

Fong, M., & Loi, N. M. (2015). The mediating role of self-compassion in student psychological health. *Australian Psychologist*, *51*(6), 431–441. doi:10.1111/ap.12185

Hall, C., Row, K. A., Wuensch, K. L., & Godley, K. R. (2013). The role of self-compassion in physical and psychological well-being. *The Journal of Psychology, 147*(4), 311–323. doi:10.1080/00223980.2012.693138 PMID:23885635

Hartley, M. T. (2011). Examining the relationships between resilience, mental health, and academic persistence in undergraduate college students. *Journal of American College Health, 59*(7), 596–604. doi:10.1080/07448481.2010.515632 PMID:21823954

Keyes, C. L. M., Kendler, K. S., Myers, J. M., & Martin, C. C. (2015). The genetic overlap and distinctiveness of flourishing and the big five personality traits. *Journal of Happiness Studies, 16*(3), 655–668. doi:10.1007/s10902-014-9527-2

Komarraju, M., Karua, S. J., & Schmeck, R. R. (2009). Role of the big five personality traits in predicting college students academic motivation and achievement. *Learning and Individual Differences, 19*(1), 47–52. doi:10.1016/j.lindif.2008.07.001

Lopez, S. J., & Sidhu, P. (2013, March). U.S. teachers love their lives, but struggle in the workplace. *Gallup*. Retrieved from http://www.gallup.com/poll/161516/teachers-love-lives-struggle-workplace.aspx

MetLife Inc. (2013). *The MetLife Survey of the American Teacher: Challenges for School Leadership*. Retrieved from https://www.metlife.com/assets/cao/foundation/MetLife-Teacher-Survey-2012.pdf

Muenks, K., Wigfield, A., Seung Yang, J., & O'Neal, C. R. (2016). How true is grit? Assessing its relations to high school and college students' personality characteristics, self-regulation, engagement, and achievement. *Journal of Educational Psychology*.

Neely, M. E., Schallert, D. L., Mohammed, S. S., Roberts, R. M., & Chen, Y. (2009). Self-kindness when facing stress: The role of self-compassion, goal regulation, and support in college students well-being. *Motivation and Emotion, 33*(1), 88–97. doi:10.1007/s11031-008-9119-8

Neff, K. D., & McGehee, P. (2010). Self-compassion and psychological resilience among adolescents and young adults. *Self and Identity, 9*(3), 225–240. doi:10.1080/15298860902979307

Park, C. L., Wright, B. R. E., Pais, J., & Ray, D. M. (2016). Daily stress and self-control. *Journal of Social and Clinical Psychology*, *25*(9), 738–753. doi:10.1521/jscp.2016.35.9.738

Parks-Leduc, L., Feldman, G., & Bardi, A. (2015). Personality traits and personal values: A meta-analysis. *Personality and Social Psychology*, *19*(1), 3–29. doi:10.1177/1088868314538548 PMID:24963077

Tangney, J. P., Baumeister, R. F., & Boone, A. L. (2004). High self-control predicts good adjustment, less pathology, better grades, and interpersonal success. *Journal of Personality*, *72*(2), 271–324. doi:10.1111/j.0022-3506.2004.00263.x PMID:15016066

Tugade, M. M., & Fredickson, B. L. (2004). Resilient individuals use positive emotions to bounce back from negative emotional experiences. *Journal of Personality and Social Psychology*, *86*(2), 320–333. doi:10.1037/0022-3514.86.2.320 PMID:14769087

Vainio, M. M., & Daukantaite, D. (2015). Grit and different aspects of well-being: Direct and indirect relationships via sense of coherence and authenticity. *Journal of Happiness Studies*, *17*(5), 2119–2147. doi:10.1007/s10902-015-9688-7

Chapter 4
Strategies for the College Classroom

Alison Puliatte
State University of New York at Plattsburgh, USA

Melissa Martin
State University of New York at Plattsburgh, USA

Jean Mockry
State University of New York at Plattsburgh, USA

Denise Simard
State University of New York at Plattsburgh, USA

Maureen E. Squires
State University of New York at Plattsburgh, USA

ABSTRACT

College students often encounter situations that may cause them to experience stress and anxiety. The students' response to these situations can impact their mental health and well-being. This chapter discusses the impact of college students' ability to regulate their emotions when faced with stressful situations. Examples of mindfulness based practices that can be integrated into a college classroom are presented as tools to help college students regulate their emotions in order to improve their mental health and well-being.

DOI: 10.4018/978-1-5225-3793-9.ch004

INTRODUCTION

In order to help college students cultivate flourishing mental health and well-being, we need to understand the role that emotions play in our ability to handle the challenges we face each day. We also need to provide students with tools to overcome stress and anxiety. While this chapter focuses on college students enrolled in teacher preparation programs, the ideas can be transferred to other disciplines. This chapter begins by exploring a model of emotional intelligence in order to develop an understanding of how we process our emotions. Next, we will examine how we are able to regulate our emotions and how this ability impacts our daily experiences. We will then review the theory and research related to mindfulness based practices which is an approach that helps us regulate our emotions. Finally, we will discuss several mindfulness based practices that can be incorporated into a college classroom to help students cope with the emotional challenges they face on a daily basis.

EMOTIONAL INTELLIGENCE

Mayer and Salovey's (1997) model of emotional intelligence identifies four mental abilities: perception of emotion, use of emotion to facilitate thought, understanding of emotion, and management of emotion. Perception of emotion refers to the ability to accurately perceive emotions in yourself and others by reading facial expressions, tone of voice and body language. "The ability to recognize one's own emotions and identify how others are feeling requires attention to multiple internal and external cues and the analysis of both verbal and nonverbal communication in oneself and others" (Brackett & Katulak, 2007, p.7). Use of emotion to facilitate thought refers to the ability to use emotions to prioritize thinking as well as to think creatively. This ability allows us to make cognitive decisions that are guided by our understanding of the emotional impact of our actions. Understanding of emotion refers to the ability to associate emotional responses with the typical actions that are associated with them. For example, it is the understanding that anger is typically associated with aggressive actions. Management of emotions refers to the ability to regulate your own as well as other's emotions in order to reach a specific goal. We will explore the idea of emotional regulation later in this chapter.

Emotional intelligence is viewed as a malleable rather than fixed trait, meaning that our level of emotional intelligence is able to increase with training. Emotional intelligence training focuses on recognizing, labeling, understanding, expressing and regulating emotions in response to situational and contextual cues (Brackett & Caruso, 2006).

Why Is Emotional Intelligence Important for Teachers?

Teaching is a stressful profession because teachers need to meet the demands of their administrators, parents, and students while trying to implement engaging lessons that are differentiated to meet the individual needs of the diverse learners in their classrooms. In addition, added pressure has been placed on teachers in recent years due to the constant changes in educational policies that impact a teachers' annual professional performance review. Given these professional requirements, combined with stress from their personal lives, it is no wonder that teachers experience anxiety and burnout. As teachers and administrators, we saw first-hand the increase in the number of teachers each year that required emotional support for overcoming the stress and anxiety they were feeling. This impacted not only the teachers, but also their students because teachers took days off of work due to emotional challenges. In addition, if they were having a difficult time managing their mental health and well-being, they were not able to be fully present for their students. An approach to helping teachers successfully face these emotional challenges is to support and enhance their emotional intelligence skills.

It is critical for teachers to have strong emotional intelligence because "teacher effectiveness is dependent upon the abilities to recognize which emotions are best for different situations, to harness emotional energy to facilitate thinking and behavior, and to generate optimal emotional states for different contexts" (Brackett & Katulak, 2007, p. 9). Teachers use their emotional intelligence abilities to positively influence "effective classroom management, stress reduction, functional professional and personal relationships, and overall quality of life" (Brackett & Katulak, 2007, p. 11). In addition, having control over emotional responses is purported to contribute to psychological balance and emotional well-being (Ramel, Goldin, Carmona, & McQuaid, 2004).

Emotions influence teachers' cognitions including their attention, memory and problem-solving ability. Positive emotions tend to have positive influences on these cognitive areas while negative emotions have negative influences.

Emotions also impact teacher motivation in the areas of intrinsic motivation, attributions, efficacy belief and goals. For example, negative emotions tend to reduce intrinsic motivation in teachers. Self-efficacy is another area that is influenced by emotions whereas; it is increased by positive moods and is decreased by negative moods. Positive emotions result in more ambitious goals that are mastery and approach goals while negative emotions are linked with performance and avoidance goals (Sutton and Wheatley, 2003).

Teachers' emotions impact how they respond to students, colleagues and parents, as well as their teaching methods. For example, if teachers are experiencing negative emotions they tend to attribute student misbehavior to "…students' laziness or deviousness, rather than real need, and are unlikely to provide the appropriate instructional or emotional support…" (Sutton & Wheatley, 2003, p. 39).

Teachers' Emotions

Teaching evokes a multitude of positive and negative emotions throughout the school day in response to the teacher's social interactions with students, parents and colleagues. In a review of literature examining teachers' emotions, Sutton and Wheatley (2003) found that teachers experience a wide variety of emotions in response to goal incongruence, factors outside the classroom, colleagues, parents, student effort, fatigue, stress, student behavior and student learning. The positive emotions reported by teachers included love, caring, joy, satisfaction, and excitement while the negative emotions reported by teachers included anger, frustration, anxiety, helplessness, guilt, and sadness.

Since emotional intelligence is critical for teachers, one would expect for it to be nurtured in pre-service teachers. Corcoran and Tormey (2012) measured the emotional intelligence of pre-service teachers to determine their ability to perceive emotions in themselves and others, use emotions to facilitate thinking, understand emotional information and manage emotion. The four areas of emotional intelligence that were measured were (1) perception, appraisal, and expression of emotion; (2) using emotions to facilitate thinking; (3) understanding and analyzing emotional information; and (4) regulating emotions. The researchers found that on average, the pre-service teachers' emotional intelligence scores were in the competent range, but they were significantly below the expected scores and norms for the wider population. In addition, females outperformed males in all measures of emotional intelligence. On average, the students' lowest scores were in the skill area of understanding and analyzing emotional information. The findings of this study are concerning because given the social nature of teaching, it is important for teachers to have high levels of emotional intelligence. The results of this study support the need to integrate activities in the college classroom to support pre-service teachers' emotional intelligence in order to prepare them to be effective teachers.

EMOTIONAL REGULATION

Serving as teachers and administrators, we have had the privilege of visiting a multitude of classrooms to work with many talented students and teachers on the elementary level. During our classroom visits we were always aware of the climate of classroom. For example, some rooms were always calm and organized, some had high energy, and some had a welcoming spirit, while others did not. It was not surprising to observe that the climate of each room mirrored the teacher's emotional state in the present moment. This was especially evident when the same group of students met with different teachers throughout the day. When the students were with a positive and warm teacher who was genuinely excited about teaching, they tended to be highly engaged in their work and they displayed positive social skills. On the other hand, when the same group of students was with a teacher who was displaying negative emotions, the students tended to be off task, unmotivated to learn and they displayed poor interpersonal skills. During these classroom visits, what was appearing to stand out was that the teacher's ability to regulate their own emotions impacted the climate of the classroom as well as their students' motivation to learn. Therefore, teachers' emotional regulation had an influence on their students' learning and development.

Even if teachers try to hide their negative emotions, students are aware of and influenced by their teachers' moods because of the physiological and physical changes that occur in response to emotional states (i.e., body language, tone of voice, facial expression, reddening of face, rate of breath, sweating). Since students are influenced by and able to identify teachers' emotions, teachers need to learn how to regulate their emotions in order to best meet their students' needs (Sutton and Wheatley, 2003).

Gross (1998) describes emotions as response tendencies whereas emotions are described by how individuals respond to situational factors. He defines emotional regulation as "the processes by which individuals influence which emotions they have, when they have them, and how they express these emotions" (Gross, 1998, p. 275). He describes five sets of emotion regulatory processes: situation selection, situation modification, attention deployment, cognitive change, and response modulation. Situation selection refers to a process to regulate emotions by which individuals approach or avoid certain situations based on their personal desires in order to elicit or avoid particular emotions. Situation modification is a process of emotional regulation by which individuals modify the situation in order to change its emotional impact. Attentional deployment is a process of emotional regulation by which individuals shift their attention away from or toward the situation at hand in an effort to regulate their emotions. Cognitive change is a process of emotional regulation that involves the individual changing the way they think about and interpret a situation in order to regulate their emotional response. Response modulation is a process of emotional regulation where the individual attempts to regulate their physiological, experiential or behavioral responses to a situation.

The five processes of emotion regulation presented by Gross (1998) provide us with a comprehensive view of the different aspects in which individuals can regulate their emotions. However, often times we are unable to regulate our emotions through situation selection and situation modification because we are unable to modify or select situations we are faced with. For example, we may be faced with unexpected situations that evoke negative emotions. Since these situations were unexpected, we do not have the opportunity to modify them or select whether or not to be faced with them. When this occurs, it is important that we have tools to help us initiate the processes of attention deployment, cognitive change, and response modulation so that we are able to regulate our own emotions. Mindfulness practices are tools that can assist us with Gross' (1998) processes of attentional deployment, cognitive change and response modulation. We will discuss details relating to mindfulness later in this chapter.

The Impact of Emotional Regulation

One's ability to regulate their emotions impacts their interpersonal interactions and relationships. In a four year longitudinal study, researchers examined the relationship between emotional regulation and social functioning in college students (English, John, Srivastava, & Gross, 2012). The results showed that students who suppressed their emotions (as shown by not expressing their emotions) had lower levels of social connectedness than peers who demonstrated cognitive reappraisal of emotions (controlling their emotions by changing the way they think about situations). Since teaching occurs in a social context (interactions between colleagues, students and parents) teachers who are able to regulate their emotions through cognitive reappraisal rather than suppression are expected to be able to form better social connections between these groups.

Positive social and emotional abilities are important skills for teachers to possess because "social and emotional competencies influence everything from teacher-student relationships to classroom management to effective instruction to teacher burnout" (Jones, Bouffard, & Weissbourd, 2013, p. 62). There are three areas of social and emotional learning (SEL): emotional processes, social/interpersonal skills, and cognitive regulation. Emotional processes include understanding and identifying feelings, emotional regulation, and empathy. Social/interpersonal skills require an understanding of social cues, having positive interpersonal skills and understanding the intent of others' behaviors. Cognitive regulation refers to executive functions such as the ability to maintain attention and focus, working memory, and impulse inhibition (Jones, Bouffard, & Weissbourd, 2013). Teachers' SEL competencies impact the quality of teacher-student relationships as well as the teachers' classroom management and organization. In addition, students learn SEL skills from observing their teachers. Therefore, teachers are models of SEL competencies for their students.

SEL competencies should be integrated in pre-service teacher preparation programs to help develop socially and emotionally competent teachers. Teachers with higher levels of SEL demonstrate more effective classroom management because, "they are likely to be more proactive, skillfully using their emotional expressions and verbal support to promote enthusiasm and enjoyment of learning and to guide and manage student behaviors" (Jennings, & Greenberg, 2009, p. 493). Teachers who are socially and emotionally competent have high self-awareness, social awareness, and emotional regulation.

Teachers' social emotional competencies can be promoted through emotional intelligence training which focuses on enhancing our ability to recognize, understand and regulate our emotions. Teachers and students can be supported to develop their SEL competencies and overcome stress through training on emotional regulation interventions that incorporate mindfulness based stress reduction techniques.

MINDFULNESS

In the past decade, mindfulness has been popularized in the media as a way of reducing stress and improving the quality of one's life. We have seen the term mindfulness appear in posts on social media, as topics of discussion in television talk shows, and in magazines all promoting the benefits of a mindfulness-based practice. But, what exactly is mindfulness and does it truly have benefits on our mental health and well-being? In this section, we will explore the definition of mindfulness, the benefits of a mindfulness-based practice and activities to promote mindfulness in the college classroom.

What Is Mindfulness?

The construct of mindfulness has been operationally defined in the literature in a variety of ways. The majority of the definitions include the idea that mindfulness is an intentional state of consciousness that promotes awareness, being fully present, and developing a nonjudgmental acceptance of what is occurring in the present moment. According to Kabat-Zinn (2003), the founder of mindfulness based stress reduction (MBSR), "mindfulness is the awareness that emerges through paying attention on purpose, in the present moment, and nonjudgmentally to the unfolding of experience moment by moment" (p. 145). Daniel J. Siegel supported this definition when he identified mindfulness as "a way of being aware of what is happening within us and around us with a clear focus of attention on moment-to-moment experience that enables us to be fully present for life" (Jennings, 2015, p. x).

Mindfulness involves three processes: forming intention, paying attention, and adjusting your attitude (Shapiro, Carlson, Astin, & Freedman, 2006). Forming intention sets the purpose for your practice by reflecting on what you would like to focus your awareness on based on your individual needs. Paying attention allows one to be fully present and attend to your thoughts and experiences in the present moment while detaching from thoughts of the past and future. Adjusting your attitude allows one to develop a nonjudgmental acceptance of your thoughts and experiences in the present moment. These three processes are at the heart of mindfulness-based practices because together, they require the practitioner to develop awareness, be fully present, and support a nonjudgmental acceptance of what is occurring in the present. Mindfulness practice is "a commitment to reside as best as one can from moment to moment in awareness with an open heart, a spacious, non-judging, non-reactive mind," (Kabat-Zinn, 2003, p.150).

Mindfulness and Emotional Regulation

Earlier in this chapter we explored the impact of our ability to regulate our emotions on our interpersonal relationships, our mental health and our well-being as well as the need for teachers to be able to regulate their emotions in the classroom. Since teachers are in the classroom with their students, they are often not able to remove themselves from a situation that may produce a negative emotion, thus it is vital that teachers learn how to regulate their emotions. As teachers, "when we master our emotions, we can harness their power to artfully orchestrate learning environments that promote prosocial behavior, engagement, and academic success" (Jennings, 2015, p.26). When teachers consciously respond rather than automatically react to situations that arouse emotional responses, their effectiveness, resilience, and enjoyment of teaching increases. As teachers model how they are able to regulate their own emotions, they are also teaching their students how to regulate their own emotions. Since emotional regulation is a skill that has direct impact on our own social interactions as well as our mental health and well-being as well as on our students', we need to strengthen our ability to regulate our emotions especially during challenging situations. Practicing mindfulness allows us to become aware of our emotions and gives us the tools needed to regulate our emotions.

Engaging in mindfulness-based practices increases one's self awareness and helps to promote reflection and self-regulation which allows one to have greater control over their emotional response to a situation (Ekman, 2004). Practicing mindfulness-based awareness activities when we experience strong emotions allows us to more effectively regulate our emotions. To be able to regulate our emotions, we must first be aware of our emotions by being able to notice and identify them as well as identify our patterns of emotional responses. When we are able to notice our emotions, we can then practice mindfulness based activities that will allow us to consciously develop a thoughtful response to the situation rather than reactively responding. This has a direct impact on students because "[c]hildren have a strong tendency to follow an adult's emotional lead." (Jennings, 2015, p. 140).

Benefits of Mindfulness

There have been numerous studies conducted that evaluate the effects of mindfulness-based practices on the mental health and well-being of children and adults. Many of the studies examined the mindfulness based stress reduction (MBSR) program developed by Kabat- Zinn (1990) while others examined interventions modeled after this program. MBSR is a structured group intervention focusing on formal training in meditation techniques such as body-scan meditation, sitting meditation, walking meditation, and Hatha Yoga (simple stretches and postures to strengthen and relax muscles). All of the activities focus on bringing mindful attention to the breath. The meditation traditionally involves focusing your attention on an object (i.e., breath, sounds, thoughts, bodily sensations, etc.) and when your attention wanders away from this object, you are to notice and acknowledge, without judgment, that your mind wandered and then bring your focus back to the object. The training consists of eight weekly group training meetings lasting 2.5 hours each meeting and one full day (6.5 hour) of training in addition to daily meditation practice outside of the training sessions. Although the practice is modeled after Buddhism, there is not a secular component to the training.

Practicing mindfulness develops resilience in response to challenges, increases emotional regulation, increases empathetic responses to others and decreases psychological distress. Relationships have been identified between practicing mindfulness and a decrease in stress, depression, and anxiety along with an increase in general well-being, compassion and self-regulation (Lomas, Medina, Ivtzan, Rupprecht, & Eiroa-Orosa, 2017). In a study examining the influences on mental health in adults, Catalino and Fredrickson (2011) found a positive relationship between levels of mindfulness and flourishing (optimal mental health). In addition, they found that people who flourish responded to daily events with greater levels of positive emotions. Therefore, it was proposed that improving mindfulness and emotional reactivity will have positive impacts on mental health status.

In additional to behavioral changes, mindfulness based training has shown to influence structures of the brain. In a study examining the impact of MBSR training in adults, changes in their brain's gray matter were examined through magnetic resonance images. The results showed structural changes in the brain after the MBSR training. Specifically, increases in gray matter in regions of the brain associated with emotional regulation, learning and memory, self-referential processing and perspective taking were noted (Hölzel, Carmody, Vangel, Congleton, Yerramsetti, Gard, & Lazar, 2011). Through the use of functional MRIs, MBSR training has also demonstrated improvement in anxiety and depression symptoms, a reduction in negative emotions and increased self-esteem in middle age participants with social anxiety disorder (Goldin and Gross, 2010).

Benefits of Mindfulness for Teachers

Mindfulness-based practices support the social contexts of a school setting by promoting compassion for oneself and others through intrapersonal and interpersonal means. Intrapersonal skills refer to the way in which we view our own personal experiences and thoughts. In order for teachers to teach and model effective social emotional learning competencies, they need to have a high level of self-awareness. This self-awareness can be developed in teachers through mindfulness-based awareness activities. Learning how to attend to our thoughts and experiences in a non-judgmental manner allows us to develop a strong sense of self which helps us to strengthen our intrapersonal skills. Mindfulness-based practices support interpersonal skills by teaching us to relate to others through "the present-moment, nonjudgmental awareness of internal processes, including thoughts, feelings, and bodily sensations" (Jennings, 2015, p.6). Improving teachers' intrapersonal and interpersonal skills through mindfulness based practices helps teachers to more effectively collaborate with their colleagues, attend to students in a positive manner and develop meaningful communication with parents and administrators.

The impact of mindfulness based practices on teachers has been examined and documented in several studies. Teachers who participated in a modified MBSR training had a decrease in psychological symptoms, burnout and emotional exhaustion and they had an increase in mindfulness and self-compassion (Flook, Goldberg, Pinger, Bonus, & Davidson, 2013). Kemeny et al. (2011) found similar results with female school teachers who participated in an eight-week meditation and emotion regulation training. The training focused on meditation practices and promoting skills in experiencing and expressing emotions in a constructive manner. The group of teachers who received training demonstrated decreased levels of self-reported depression, anxiety, negative trait effect and trait rumination and increased levels of mindfulness and compassion. Physiological changes were observed as well where participants who practiced meditation had lower blood pressure readings when exposed to tasks that typically induce stress.

Benefits of Mindfulness for College Students

As teachers of college students who are pre-service teachers, we frequently observe that many of our students experience similar emotional struggles as in-service teachers. Students share stories about their therapy pets for their anxiety as well as visits to therapists for help with handling stress and anxiety. In seeing the similarities between pre-service and in-service teachers as well as our observations that unregulated emotional struggles have a negative impact on students, we realized that there is a great need to support our pre-service teachers' mental health and well-being now so that when they become teachers, they will have the emotional tools they need to face the stress that is present in their profession.

Mindfulness based practices can be used as a tool to address the issues facing college students today because college students who participate in mindfulness-based practices have demonstrated improvements in both their mental and physical health (Lomas, Medina, Ivtzan, Rupprecht, & Eiroa-Orosa, 2017; Murphy, Mermelstein, Edwards, & Gidycz, 2012). For example, MBSR has been found to reduce psychological distress, stress, depression and anxiety in college students; as well as increase empathy, sense of control and spiritual experiences (Astin, 1997; Shapiro, Schwartz, & Bonner, 1998; Oman, Shapiro, Thoresen, Plante, & Flinders, 2008). Bamber and Schneider (2016) found significant decreases in anxiety and stress and increases in mindfulness for college students who participated in mindfulness interventions. The researchers recommend incorporating mindfulness interventions in colleges to help students cope with the stress associated with college life. They suggest offering mindfulness training during orientation activities and also integrating activities into courses such as beginning each course with a brief mediation session.

In addition to improving the students' mental and physical health, teaching pre-service teachers to be mindful will help to prepare them for the emotional demands of their future careers as teachers. It will also give them tools to model effective emotional regulation for their future students. The interpersonal skills that are strengthened by mindfulness practices help college students to navigate complex social demands such as being away from home for the first time, interacting with new peers and working collaboratively with their classmates through group work activities. Mindfulness based practices help students with their interpersonal skills by teaching them to listen and accept other's experiences and ideas without judgment. This is a skill that is particularly useful to in-service teachers who interact with students, parents, colleagues and administrators on a daily basis. Being able to effectively listen to others without judgment allows teachers to develop positive and productive relationships that ultimately benefit the children they serve.

A variety of models of mindfulness based practices modeled after MBSR have been implemented with college students. The models have variations in implementation procedures, but they all follow the basic tenants of MBSR. For example, Caldwell, Harrison, Adams, Quin, and Greeson (2010) examined the effects of movement based courses which promote mind-body awareness on college students. Participants in the movement based courses had increased level of mindfulness which was associated with improved mood, perceived stress and sleep quality.

Koru training is a mindfulness program designed specifically for emerging adults (late teens through twenties) which differs from traditional MBSR trainings in that the training has a shorter time commitment. Koru was developed for college students by a psychiatrist and medical doctor at Duke University when they observed that traditional mindfulness programs were not sustaining the attention and interest of college students. Koru is taught in a group setting for four weeks with one 75-minute session per week. In addition, participants complete ten-minute daily meditation practices and a daily meditation log. Undergraduate, graduate, and professional students who received Koru training had a decrease in perceived stress and an increase in overall sleep quality, mindfulness and self-compassion (Greeson, Juberg, Maytan, James, & Rogers, 2014). These results are promising because positive effects on mental health were found with an intervention that is not at long as the traditional MBSR program. A shorter training program may attract college students who already feel overwhelmed with trying to manage their coursework requirement in a limited timeframe.

In addition to positive effects on mental health and well-being, mindfulness-based practices have been found to improve the physical health of college students. In a study of female college students, Murphy, Mermelstein, Edwards, and Gidycz (2012) found positive correlations between participants' levels of dispositional mindfulness and healthier eating practices, better quality of sleep and better physical health above and beyond the contribution of traditional health habits. The researchers recommend that colleges incorporate mindfulness training in order to support students' physical health.

From examining the extensive body of research on mindfulness-based practices, it is evident that there are significant positive effects on the mental and physical health of individuals who participate in mindfulness-based practices. As the literature suggests, the benefits of mindfulness-based practices are present in college students as well as professionals in a variety of fields. Since most teachers "received little if any explicit pre-service or in-service training aimed at our own personal development" (Jennings, 2015, p. 38), it is critical that we integrate these practices into our pre-service teacher preparation programs in order to provide our college students with tools that will not only help them successfully face the emotional challenges of college life, but will also prepare them to respond in a focused, non-judgmental and effective manner to the challenges they will face as teachers. "Devoting adequate time and attention to fostering such emotional awareness is extremely important in optimizing teacher effectiveness in multiple domains" (Brackett & Katulak, 2007, p. 7).

The next section introduces mindfulness-based activities that can be integrated into the college classroom. While a full MBSR training would benefit college students, not all colleges are equipped to offer such an intensive program. Instead, we suggest the idea of introducing the activities during the students' regular class time. The benefit of this design is that many of the activities only take a few minutes to teach and practice, therefore they do not interfere with the content goals of the course. Also, by repeatedly practicing these activities across a variety of settings (such as several courses) the benefits of the practice are strengthened and likely to be maintained over time.

ACTIVITIES FOR THE COLLEGE CLASSROOM

Activities which promote positive mental health and well-being that can be incorporated into a college classroom teach emotional regulation through mindfulness-based practices. The goal of such activities is to help students develop an intentional state of consciousness that promotes awareness, being fully present, and a nonjudgmental acceptance of what is occurring in the present. The practices should focus on bringing awareness to the connection between the mind and body which can be accomplished through formal and informal meditation as well as physical activities that connect movement to the breath.

College students benefit from practices that encourage daily and long-term commitment because mindfulness "develops over time, and it is greatly enhanced through regular disciplined practice, both formally and informally, on a daily basis" (Kabat-Zinn, 2003, p. 148). Mindfulness practices require awareness of our inner body perceptions such as being aware of how our body physically responds (i.e. increased heartbeat, clenched jaw) to stimuli as well as awareness of the content of our conceptual mind, our inner thoughts, beliefs, and biases (Siegel, 2010).

In order to effectively teach mindfulness based practices, instructors need to be committed to the value of the practice and should regularly participate in mindfulness based activities. It is essential that instructors have a well-established personal practice because mindfulness "cannot be taught to others in an authentic way without the instructor practicing it in his or her own life" (Kabat-Zinn, 2003, p. 149).

Mindfulness practices range from "formal practices that are undertaken for varying periods of time on a regular basis to informal practices that are aimed at cultivating a continuity of awareness in all activities of daily living" (Kabat-Zinn, 2003, p. 147). Formal mindful awareness practices include sitting meditation and contemplative movement activities. There are two forms of sitting meditation: focused attention and open monitoring. Focused attention involves "bringing mindful awareness to a particular target, such as breath, and working toward maintaining focused attention on the target" (Jennings, 2015, p. 3). To begin a focused attention practice, you sit comfortably and place all of your attention on a target, such as your breath. When your attention drifts away from your breath, nonjudgmentally recognize that your attention drifted then bring attention back to your breath. The second type of sitting meditation is open monitoring which is similar to focused attention in that you sit comfortably. However, rather than focusing your attention on a target, you monitor everything that is in your current experience. Open monitoring involves noticing all that you are experiencing through your thoughts and senses in the present moment. You become aware of these experiences, accept them and do not add judgment to them. Contemplative movement activities have the same intentions as sitting meditations because they connect your mind and body, but they incorporate movement. Examples of contemplative movement activities include yoga and tai chi.

Informal mindful awareness practices involve being attentive, aware and accepting of everything that is occurring in the present moment. During informal practice, we pause to shift our attention to become aware of the present moment without adding judgment to what we are experiencing. Informal practices do not require us to sit quietly; instead, informal practices can be initiated at any time. It is a matter of being able to stop and become aware of all that is occurring around you and being aware of how your thoughts are impacting your experience. Students of mindfulness need to first establish a solid formal practice before being able to engage in informal practices successfully. The benefit of informal practices is that at any moment when an individual is feeling overwhelmed, they can bring their thoughts back to the present moment to gain more control of their mind and body.

The practices that follow are examples of activities that can be integrated in the college classroom to promote a mindfulness practice. The goal is to strengthen college students' mental health and well-being by giving them the tools to regulate their emotions and to be aware of their thoughts and actions, as well as those of others, in a nonjudgmental way. To gain the most benefits out of any mindfulness practice, the exercises should be practiced daily. Students can be taught different types of exercises in the classroom and then should be encouraged to develop their own routine for implementing the practices on a daily basis during a time that best fits their schedule. The goal is to have students practice the exercises on a daily basis, but it should not be treated as an assignment with a grade attached because the purpose is to have the students see and feel the benefits of a regular practice which will intrinsically motivate them to continue their practice. Assigning the practices as a course requirement runs the risk of having the students view the practice as an assignment to complete rather than a life practice to embrace. The practices that follow are adapted from ideas presented and developed by Kabat-Zinn (1990, 2003) and Jennings (2015).

Setting Intention

The activity of setting intention helps students to set a purpose for their day and reminds them to make purposeful decisions that address the intention they set. Students should set their intention for the day, focus their attention on it after it is made and then reflect on their daily intention throughout the day. The process of setting intention is a personal undertaking which focuses on what is important to each individual. In order to set an intention, students need to first be reflective and determine what they would like to personally work on. It is helpful for students to write their intention for the day in a notebook that they carry throughout the day so that they can remind themselves of the intention they set.

An example of an intention that was created by a student is to be less critical of his own personal actions throughout the day. This student was working on his self-esteem and noticed that he was engaging in negative self-talk based on the judgments he was making of himself. He set his intention for the day to become aware of when he began engaging in negative self-talk. Bringing a sense of awareness to his actions allowed him to identify when he was being judgmental of himself and reminded him to accept his thoughts and actions in a nonjudgmental manner. The practice of setting this attention allowed the student to become more accepting of himself and it improved his confidence.

Three Breaths

A simple technique that can be used to teach students to be attentive to their emotions and to help regulate their physiological reactions to stress is the three breaths exercise. This is a basic breathing technique that helps to calm the nervous system. The exercise teaches students to breathe with their diaphragm while taking three slow, deep breaths. This is an exercise that can be taught in the classroom in a few minutes and students should be encouraged to utilize this technique during hectic moments.

The exercise begins with the students sitting with both feet on the floor and hands on their laps. Another variation is to have the students stand with both feet flat on the floor and hands at their sides. The students are invited to close their eyes and take a deep breath in to the count of five and then exhale to the count of five. This is repeated for three breaths. Students are reminded to focus their attention on their breath throughout the exercise.

The three breaths exercise is particularly helpful when students are faced with a situation that is causing stress. For example, students can take three breaths to help them calm down and focus before a test, before they give a presentation and when they are faced with making a difficult decision.

After this exercise was presented to a group of college students, one student implemented it with an elementary student she was working with and had positive results. The elementary student was arguing with his friends and began to get upset and angry. The college student took the elementary student to the side and had him practice the three breaths activity. This deep breathing practice calmed the elementary student down and allowed him to have a productive conversation with his peers.

Open Monitoring

Open monitoring can be practiced after you have experience with a focused attention practice. Open monitoring differs from focused attention because it calls us to bring our attention to the present moment without focusing on a specific object. This practice involves being aware of the full context of your experience in a nonjudgmental manner. It is as if you remove yourself from your thoughts and observe everything that is occurring in the present moment while being aware of how you are physically and emotionally reacting to the experience. This practice helps students to be focused and attentive in a calm manner to everything that is happening in the present moment.

To begin an open monitoring practice, first focus on your breath to help your mind settle for about 5-10 minutes. Then, turn your attention away from your breath and become aware of everything in the present moment without focusing on anything in particular. You should notice your thoughts and surroundings but do not focus on them. If you find that you become focused on a thought, "notice that your attention has been captured, name what grabbed your attention, and then loosen your mind back to open awareness" (Jennings, 2015, p. 47). If you have difficulty broadening your awareness, you can always bring your attention back to your breath to help your mind settle.

Emotion Journal

Students can be taught to keep a journal to record their emotions to help them understand their emotional responses to different situations. Developing an understanding of emotional responses helps students to regulate their emotions when they encounter situations that may arouse their emotions. Keeping an emotion journal will also help students to identify patterns of their emotional responses. Identifying patterns to emotional responses will help students to be able to have better control of regulating their emotions when faced with new and challenging situations.

The journal should include a description of the situation, how the student felt physically during the situation, the thoughts they had during the situation, and their emotional response. This activity can be incorporated into a college classroom at the beginning of class as a "do now" activity or at the end of class as an "exit slip." Students can be asked to think about a situation that recently occurred in their lives and record their emotions in response to the situation. After several days of completing journal entries, students can be asked to review their writings to find any patterns of behavior. Students can then record the patterns they identified and use this information to set an intention for the next day.

Positivity Journal

In addition to an emotion journal, students can be introduced to a positivity journal where they focus on the positive feelings they felt during day. Journal entries should include the situations that cultivated the positive feeling as well as the impact the positive feeling had on the student's day. Similar to an emotion journal, students can write entries in their positivity journal at the start or end of class and they should be encouraged to continue this practice outside of class time as well. This journal helps students regulate their emotions because becoming mindfully aware of positive feelings helps to generate a positive response to future situations.

Body Scan

The body scan practice allows students to identify their emotions and physical sensations as well as bring themselves into the present moment by directing their attention to different parts of their body. The practice helps students to identify areas of the body where they are holding tension and to use their breath to relax these areas. In addition, the body scan helps to focus attention and awareness on the connection between the mind and body.

This practice is most effective when it is done lying down. While this may not be practical in a classroom, the practice can be introduced in a sitting position and the students can be encouraged to engage in the practice outside of class time when they can lay down. The practice begins by bringing attention to your breath until your mind settles. Next, you bring your attention to your feet to notice any sensations you have there with the purpose of becoming aware of the sensations you feel. You repeat this activity throughout your body moving from your feet to calves, knees, thighs, back of your torso, shoulders, front of your torso, neck and finally your head. As you complete the body scan, bring attention to your entire body and if there is an area where you still feel tension, direct your awareness back to this area. You end the practice by bringing awareness back to your breath.

Centering

The practice of centering is another example of an exercise that can be incorporated into a college classroom with minimal interruption to the course. Centering is helpful to students when they feel like their energy is scattered because it helps to make them feel grounded and centered in the present moment. This practice involves standing with your feet shoulder width apart. Next, focus your attention on the center of your core which is a few inches below your naval and an inch into your body. Spend a few minutes focusing on this part of your body, which is the center of gravity of your body, until you feel grounded and less scattered.

Mindful Walking

Mindful walking is a form of walking meditation where the student practices focusing their attention on the act of walking. The purpose of this activity is to help the student pay attention to the present moment by focusing on breathing and movement. The goal is to have the student become more aware of themselves in the present moment rather than focusing on the past or future events.

Mindful walking begins with taking a few minutes to practice centering. Once you feel centered, begin to slowly walk while focusing your attention to the soles of your feet. As you walk, fix your attention on the soles of your feet noticing the sensations you feel as your weight shifts throughout your feet. Continue this walking exercise focusing your attention on the soles of your feet.

Mindful Listening

Mindful listening is a critical skill that needs to be developed in college students. The ability to actively listen helps to improve interpersonal interactions and allows us to be fully present in a conversation rather than thinking about what we are going to say in response to the speaker. When we listen for the sake of understanding the speaker rather than for the sake of responding, we are able to develop deeper connections with others. During a mindful listening exercise, students should be taught to "notice the sound of the other person's voice- the tone, the volume and so forth. We notice the other's facial expressions, and we listen to her or his words without automatically judging them and reacting to them. At the same time we notice our internal experience-our thoughts and feelings-without judgment" (Jennings, 2015, p. 121).

Mindful listening can be practiced by ringing a chime and focusing your listening to the sound until the ringing ends. This practice can be used to help focus your attention at the beginning of a mindfulness activity. Another activity to practice mindful listening is to have students work with a partner to discuss a selected topic. The students are given a set amount of time to take turns talking about the topic. One student begins speaking while their partner listens without responding. When the time is up, the partner who was listening paraphrases what their partner said and discusses how their partner felt about the topic based on their physical responses (tone of voice, body language, facial expressions, etc.). This activity requires the student who was listening to focus in on what their partner was saying as well as the nonverbal cues they were presenting. This encourages the listener to be present and focused throughout the conversation rather than thinking about how they are going to respond or letting their thoughts wander.

CONCLUSION

College students are faced with experiences that can cause them to feel overcome by stress and anxiety on a regular basis. The pressures of meeting deadlines for course assignments, handling relationship issues, managing a job while being a student, and trying to make the transition from teenager to young adult are a few examples of situations that can feel overwhelming and may cause students to feel anxious. Since many of these situations cannot be avoided or even controlled, students need to acquire strategies for developing resiliency when faced with stressful situations. The mindfulness based practices presented in this chapter are examples of tools that students can use to help regulate their emotional responses when faced with challenging situations. In addition, the practices help students stay present and focused in a nonjudgmental manner which will help them to develop positive mental health and well-being.

The next chapter, *Campus-Wide Initiatives*, discusses how institutes of higher education can support mindfulness based practices through training for faculty and staff and by developing a college-wide focus aimed at addressing the mental health and well-being needs of college students. The final chapter, *What is Next: Future Considerations*, addresses the challenges of implementing mindfulness based practices in a college setting.

REFERENCES

Astin, J.A. (1997). Stress reduction through mindfulness meditation: Effects on psychological symptomatology, sense of control, and spiritual experiences. *Psychotherapy and Psychosomatics*, *66*, 97–106. doi:10.1159/000289116 PMID:9097338

Bamber, M. D., & Schneider, J. K. (2016). Mindfulness-based meditation to decrease stress and anxiety in college students: A narrative synthesis of the research. *Educational Research Review, 18*, 1–32. doi:10.1016/j.edurev.2015.12.004

Brackett, M. A., & Caruso, D. R. (2006). *The emotionally intelligent teacher*. Ann Arbor, MI: Quest Education.

Brackett, M. A., & Katulak, N. (2007). The emotionally intelligent classroom: Skill-based training for teachers and students. In J. Ciarrochi & J. D. Mayer (Eds.), *Improving emotional intelligence: A practitioner's guide* (pp. 1–27). New York, NY: Psychology Press/Taylor & Francis.

Caldwell, C., Harrison, M., Adams, M., Quin, R., & Greeson, J. (2010). Developing mindfulness in college students through movement based courses: Effects on self-regulatory self-*efficacy, mood, stress and sleep quality. Journal of American College Health, 58*(8), 433–442. doi:10.1080/07448480903540481 PMID:20304755

Catalino, L. I., & Fredrickson, B. L. (2011). A Tuesday in the life of a flourisher: The role of positive emotional reactivity in optimal mental health. *Emotion (Washington, D.C.), 11*(4), 938–950. doi:10.1037/a0024889 PMID:21859208

Corcoran, R. P., & Tormey, R. (2012). How emotionally intelligent are pre-service teachers? *Teaching and Teacher Education, 28*(5), 750–759. doi:10.1016/j.tate.2012.02.007

Ekman, P. (2004). *Emotions revealed* (2nd ed.). New York: Times Books.

English, T., John, O. P., Srivastava, S., & Gross, J. J. (2012). Emotion regulation and peer-rated social functioning: A four-year longitudinal study. *Journal of Research in Personality, 46*(6), 780–784. doi:10.1016/j.jrp.2012.09.006 PMID:23471162

Flook, L., Goldberg, S. B., Pinger, L., Bonus, K., & Davidson, R. J. (2013). Mindfulness for teachers: A pilot study to assess effects on stress, burnout and teaching efficacy. *Mind, Brain, and Education, 7*(3), 1–22. doi:10.1111/mbe.12026 PMID:24324528

Goldin, P. R., & Gross, J. J. (2010). Effects of mindfulness-based stress reduction on emotion regulation in social anxiety disorder. *Emotion (Washington, D.C.), 10*(1), 83–91. doi:10.1037/a0018441 PMID:20141305

Greeson, J. M., Juberg, M. K., Maytan, M., James, K., & Rogers, H. (2014). A randomized controlled trial of Koru: A mindfulness program for college students and other emerging adults. *Journal of American College Health, 62*(4), 222–233. doi:10.1080/07448481.2014.887571 PMID:24499130

Gross, J. J. (1998). The emerging field of emotion regulation: An integrative review. *Review of General Psychology, 2*(3), 271–299. doi:10.1037/1089-2680.2.3.271

Hölzel, B. K., Carmody, J., Vangel, M., Congleton, C., Yerramsetti, S. M., Gard, T., & Lazar, S. W. (2011). Mindfulness practice leads to increases in regional brain gray matter density. *Psychiatry Research: Neuroimaging, 191*(1), 36–43. doi:10.1016/j.pscychresns.2010.08.006 PMID:21071182

Jennings, P. A. (2015). *Mindfulness for teachers: Simple skills for peace and productivity in the classroom.* NY, NY: W.W. Norton & Company, Inc.

Jennings, P. A., & Greenberg, M. T. (2009). The prosocial classroom: Teacher social and emotional competence in relation to student and classroom outcomes. *Review of Educational Research, 79*(1), 491–525. doi:10.3102/0034654308325693

Jones, S. M., Bouffard, S. M., & Weissbourd, R. (2013). Educators social and emotional skills vital to learning. *Kappan, 94*(8), 62–65. doi:10.1177/003172171309400815

Kabat-Zinn, J. (1990). *Full catastrophe living: Using the wisdom of your body and mind to face stress, pain and illness.* New York: Dell Publishing.

Kabat-Zinn, J. (2003). Mindfulness-based interventions in context: Past, present, and future. *Clinical Psychology: Science and Practice, 10*(2), 144–156. doi:10.1093/clipsy.bpg016

Kemeny, M. E., Foltz, C., Cavanagh, J. F., Cullen, M., Giese-Davis, J., Jennings, P., & Ekman, P. et al. (2011). Contemplative/emotion training reduces negative emotional behavior and promotes prosocial responses. *Emotion.* PMID:22148989

Lomas, T., Medina, J. C., Ivtzan, I., Rupprecht, S., & Eiroa-Orosa, F. J. (2017). The impact of mindfulness on the wellbeing and performance of educators: A systematic review of the empirical literature. *Teaching and Teacher Education, 61*, 132–141. doi:10.1016/j.tate.2016.10.008

Mayer, J. D., & Salovey, P. (1997). What is emotional intelligence? In P. Salovey & D. J. Sluyter (Eds.), *Emotional Development and Emotional Intelligence: Educational Implications* (pp. 3–34). New York, NY: Basic Books, Inc.

Murphy, M. J., Mermelstein, L. C., Edwards, K. M., & Gidycz, C. A. (2012). The benefits of dispositional mindfulness in physical health: A longitudinal study of female college students. *Journal of American College Health*, *60*(5), 341–348. doi:10.1080/07448481.2011.629260 PMID:22686356

Oman, D. O., Shapiro, S. L., Thoresen, C. E., Plante, T. G., & Flinders, T. (2008). Meditation lowers stress and supports forgiveness among college students: A randomized controlled trial. *Journal of American College Health*, *56*(5), 569–578. doi:10.3200/JACH.56.5.569-578 PMID:18400671

Ramel, W., Goldin, P. R., Carmona, P. E., & McQuaid, J. R. (2004). The effects of mindfulness meditation on cognitive processes and affect in patients with past depression. *Cognitive Therapy and Research*, *28*(4), 433–455. doi:10.1023/B:COTR.0000045557.15923.96

Shapiro, S. L., Schwartz, G. E., & Bonner, G. (1998). Effects of mindfulness-based stress reduction on medical and premedical students. *Journal of Behavioral Medicine*, *21*(6), 581–599. doi:10.1023/A:1018700829825 PMID:9891256

Sutton, R., & Wheatley, K. F. (2003). Teachers emotions and teaching: A review of the literature and directions for future research. *Educational Psychology Review*, *15*(4), 327–358. doi:10.1023/A:1026131715856

Chapter 5
Campus-Wide Initiatives

Maureen E. Squires
State University of New York at Plattsburgh, USA

Melissa Martin
State University of New York at Plattsburgh, USA

Jean Mockry
State University of New York at Plattsburgh, USA

Alison Puliatte
State University of New York at Plattsburgh, USA

Denise Simard
State University of New York at Plattsburgh, USA

ABSTRACT

In this chapter, the authors situate mental health issues in the context of U.S. institutes of higher education. They provide a brief history of the provision of mental health services on campus and contends that postsecondary schools should shift to a campus-wide, preventive, proactive approach to promote student flourishing. Four specific areas for interventions are discussed. These include academic or curricular adjustments, increased awareness and knowledge, supportive environments, and appropriate policies and procedures. These initiatives (which are not only the responsibility of "experts") rely on the open communication and collaboration of all members of the campus community.

DOI: 10.4018/978-1-5225-3793-9.ch005

INTRODUCTION

The authors begin by providing a brief history of the provision of mental health services on campus. Then they discuss four areas in which campus-wide initiatives have been found effective in supporting the mental health of college students. These include curricular adjustments, community environments, mental health literacy, and campus policy. These focus areas have been selected as they are most applicable to this audience: college/university faculty and staff whose background are not necessarily in mental health. These are the professionals who will have regular contact with students, those with and without mental health issues. As such, the initiatives in this chapter can be understood and implemented by professionals without degrees in the mental health field.

OVERVIEW

With the increasing prevalence of mental illness in institutes of higher education (IHE), research suggests that colleges and universities must adapt to better serve their students. Reactive approaches and individualized counseling alone are not sufficient. Moreover, compartmentalized service (where responsibility for college student mental health resides in counseling centers) has limited influence. It is recommended that IHE shift from a targeted focus to a campus-wide focus and direct their efforts toward preventive measures (Fink, 2014; Hartley, 2012; Swaner, 2007; Wood, 2012). In the past few decades several organizations have proposed ways to facilitate this transition.

The Jed Foundation (JED), though not the only organization aimed at promoting emotional and mental well-being, is a leader in this field. It offers support to schools, students, families, and communities to strengthen mental health. JED's 7-point Strategic Plan is comprehensive, attending to the following areas: developing life skills, promoting social connectedness, identifying students at risk, increasing help-seeking behavior, providing substance abuse and mental health services, following crisis management procedures, and restricting access to potentially lethal means (JED, 2016). Such an approach affects multiple levels of the campus community from college policy, to particular organizations like student mental health services, to faculty training and involvement, to curriculum design, to student enculturation.

Building on the recommendations of JED and other relevant literature, IHE can take multiple steps to improve the mental health of college students. Academic adjustments to face-to-face and online courses have been found to mediate the negative effects of stress in academic settings. Such curricular changes include engaged learning models and course offerings in mental well-being (DiPlacito-DeRango, 2016; Fink, 2014; Mitchell, Darrow, Haggerty, & Neill, 2012; Savini, 2016; Swaner, 2007). IHE that endorse social and academic inclusion via residential communities, campus activities, and learning communities are found to be more supportive and promote a sense of student belonging, which are favorable factors of mental health (Condra, Dineen, Gauthier, Gills, Jack-Davies, & Condra, 2015; Fink, 2014). Moreover, IHE at all levels (leadership, faculty, support staff, and students) must be fully aware and fully trained to promote resilience and identify signs of mental illness (Barr, 2014; Condra et al., 2015; Hartley, 2012, Wood, 2010) to create environments in which students can flourish. Additionally, campuses should have the necessary policies and procedures in place to promote well-being and intervene when students are in mental distress (Condra et al., 2015; DiPlacito-DeRango, 2016; Murphy & Baines, 2015; Silverman, 2008; Wood, 2012).

PROVISION OF MENTAL HEALTH SERVICES ON CAMPUS

In the United States, the provision of mental health services in IHE morphed considerably during the 20th century. Amherst College is credited with establishing the first student health services in 1861, yet the first mental health services was not established until 1910 by Princeton University (Kraft, 2009; Kraft, 2011). In the first half of the 20th century, college mental health services were developed and primarily provided by psychiatrists. As the field grew, clinical psychologists and psychiatric social workers began providing services as part of a multidisciplinary team approach (Kraft, 2009; Kraft, 2011). Yet, services were often split between two departments: psychiatric mental health and other counseling resources. This model was expanded mid-century when increasing numbers of students, funded by the GI bill, entered colleges and universities (Kraft, 2009; Kraft, 2011). Increased student enrollment necessitated increased health professionals on campus. It also meant providing a broader range of services to address the new needs of students. Similarly, it required a new service-delivery approach.

A shift occurred mid-century. Mental health services no longer focused solely on the "mental hygiene" of a few acute students receiving in-patient care (Kraft, 2009; Kraft, 2011). Mental health services began to have a broader purpose, serving a larger population and doing so through ambulatory care services (Kraft, 2009; Kraft, 2011). These services included career or vocational counseling, psychotherapy, medication assists, and consultation across campus. In the second half of the century, another shift occurred (Kraft, 2009; Kraft, 2011). Campus counseling centers had a growing and changing role in the provision of mental health services moving from that of "providing only direct counseling services to one that makes multiple contributions to a campus community" (Bishop, 2010, p. 249). Addressing the ever-changing needs of college students, mental health services expanded their scope to deal with drug and alcohol abuse (initiated in the '70s), public health issues (initiated in the '80s), and recently stress, anxiety, and depression. Additionally, prevention efforts and education campaigns are now a significant part of mental health services.

Today's mental health services on campus are geared toward a diverse population and intended to be proactive rather than reactive. Standards set forth by the International Association of Counseling Services (IACS) support a systemic and comprehensive campus initiative. It highlights four key functions of campus counseling services: "individual and group student counseling; prevention and outreach; consultation to faculty and staff; and contributions to campus safety" (Prince, 2015, p. 6). These standards suggest that campus counseling services are important, though not the sole factor influencing student mental health. Faculty and staff also play an essential role. Moreover, these standards indicate that mental health services do not reside in a single location on campus. This notion is echoed by Bishop (2010). In reviewing the literature, Bishop (2010) found a continued need for counseling centers to make clear their engagement in "outreach, programming, and consultation work" (p. 250), implying that mental health services in IHE are most effective when viewed as a shared responsibility.

The responsibility of college student mental health does not reside within a single department or office. It is the responsibility of the entire campus community. Many IHE have adopted a "public mental health model – a model that attempts to address environmental factors of the campus that influence students' mental health" (Prince, 2015, p. 7). Through such a paradigm, members of student affairs and student services, faculty, staff, and students themselves work together to improve well-being on campus. It has been argued that colleges and universities are well situated to have a positive effect on mental health. Postsecondary education is often the place where:

A single integrated setting encompasses their [students'] main activities – both career related and social – as well as health services and other support services. Campuses, by their scholarly nature, are also well positioned to develop, evaluate, and disseminate best practices. In short, colleges offer a unique opportunity to address one of the most significant public health problems among late adolescents and young adults. (Hunt & Eisenberg, 2010, p. 3)

Hence, the focus of this chapter: college-wide initiatives that can enhance student mental well-being.

COMPREHENSIVE INTERVENTIONS

There are multiple ways in which IHE can support the mental health of college students. This section of the chapter focuses on building a sense of community, increasing awareness and knowledge, curriculum adjustments, and establishing campus-wide policy. Although psychotherapy and medications can be used to treat some students, they are not discussed here. Likewise, interventions for students with mental health illnesses requiring individual care from the Counseling Center and/or private mental health providers (e.g., psychologists, clinical social workers, certified counselors, licensed nurse psychotherapists, or psychiatrists) are not discussed here. As a teacher educator, such therapies fall outside of my purview. Moreover, my intent is to present strategies that can apply to many students, not simply those requiring intensive or prolonged care, and that can be used preventatively.

Building a Sense of Community to Promote Mental Health

Mental health, or flourishing, does not simply exist in the absence of mental illness. As Keyes (2005 & 2007) describes in his model of Mental Health as Flourishing, there are 13 factors associated with flourishing. These include positive affect and avowed quality of life (emotional well-being); self-acceptance, personal growth, purpose in life, environmental mastery, autonomy, and positive relations with others (psychological well-being); and social acceptance, social actualization, social contribution, social coherence, and social integration (social well-being) (Keyes, 2007). In replicating Keyes' work, Fink (2014) obtained similar findings. His analysis revealed four significant predictors of college student mental health. These include a supportive college environment, a sense of belonging, professional confidence, and civic engagement (Fink, 2014). Fink (2014) concluded that "socially supportive climates, such as easy transitions into college and supportive residence halls, as well as intermediate outcomes such as sense of belonging" were particularly strong predictors (p. 386). Myriad other researchers have noted similar associations with college student mental health, focusing especially on the type of environment in which students live and learn.

Without oversimplifying IHE, I conceptualize campuses as on a continuum from "cool" to "warm" with various degrees in between. Cool campuses are those that lack a sense of community and promote a sense of isolation. These are the campuses that have a "non-accepting culture" (Tinklin, Riddell, & Wilson, 2005, p. 507). As such, differences are viewed as deficiencies rather than natural occurrences that warrant empathy, compassion, and accommodation. On cool campuses public and personal stigma are prevalent.

Public, or social, stigma "is characterized by prejudicial attitudes and discriminating behaviour directed towards individuals with mental health problems as a result of the psychiatric label they have been given" (Davey, 2013, p. 1). In other words, it is the stigma of others (family members, friends, instructors, and the media) emanating from outside the individual with the mental health disorder. Public stigma can present as "prejudicial attitudes and discriminating behavior" (Davey, 2013, p. 2). Stereotypes of individuals with mental health disorders as dangerous or intellectually inferior can lead to social isolation and lowered expectations. Personal stigma is just as, if not more, detrimental.

Self-stigma, also known as perceived stigma, "is the internalizing by the mental health sufferer of their perceptions of discrimination" (Davey, 2013, p. 1). It occurs when the individual with mental illness believes the negative stereotypes ascribed to his/her psychiatric label. Self-stigma may result in feelings of fear and shame (Condra et al., 2015; Davey, 2013; Tucker, Hammer, Vogel, Bitman, Wade, & Maier, 2013), exacerbate symptoms of the disability (Pedersen & Paves, 2014), and heighten social isolation (Pedersen & Paves, 2014; Tinklin et al., 2005; Tucker et al., 2013). Stigma is a chief concern as it has been identified as a barrier to college students seeking help for mental illness (DiPlacito-DeRango, 2016; Hunt & Eisenberg, 2010; Pedersen & Paves, 2014; Shatkin, Diamond, Zhao, DiMeglio, Chodaczek, & Bruzzese, 2016). It can affect students' self-concept and influence their perceived need for help or their likelihood to deal with mental illness on their own.

On the contrary, warm campuses are defined by their open and accepting nature. Here, differences are not considered flaws. Rather, diversity is anticipated and welcomed. Moreover, pro-social interactions are encourage and fostered so that students do not feel a sense of alienation. Such environments are known as "welcoming culture[s]" (Condra et al., 2015, p. 277) supported by a "web of caring" (Asidao & Sevig, 2014, p. 132) and "social networks that reinforce a sense of campus community" (Silverman, 2008). In this way the camps is ecological in nature, where human beings interact with each other and with their environment. Interactions on warm campuses are different from interactions on cool campuses. They are grounded in compassion and empathy for others. Summarizing Kuh, Swaner (2007) underscores the importance of:

Small, 'human-scale' environments [that] encourage responsible, health-enhancing behavior," and emphasizes that where faculty and student contact is frequent and classes are small, "a college or university encourages its members to know each other, a precursor to caring for one another. (p. 21)

I would go farther, suggesting that positive interactions are not limited to those between students or among students and faculty. Positive interactions include all members of the campus community. This highlights the value of positive, supportive relationships grounded in getting to know and understand others.

Such warm campuses can be fostered in academic and non-academic settings. In fact, many researchers suggest that a comprehensive focus best serves college students. Classrooms can be turned into learning communities where students are engaged in meaningful ways and where students work with one another to grow intellectually and empathically (Bertram, 2010; Fink, 2014; Wrench, Garrett, & King, 2013). Residence halls, where students live in close proximity to a great number of diverse peers, are prime places to develop inclusive spaces (Bertram, 2010; Fink, 2014). Social networks and friendships are a critical component of warm campuses (Bertram, 2010; Fink, 2014; Wrench et al., 2013). Such relationships may start in the residential communities and typically expand beyond the dorm. Events and activities (academic, social, athletic, club-related, Greek life-based) can support the development of peer relationships, which shape the campus community. In addition to peer relationships, student-faculty relationships can contribute to a welcoming environment. Positive student-faculty relationships occur both inside and outside the classroom. One way to enhance such openness is to schedule events where faculty and students interact informally (Quinn, Wilson, MacIntyre, & Tinklin, 2009). In each of these ways, members of the campus gather to get to know each other and begin to form a community.

By definition, a community includes myriad individuals unified by common interests. This can include persons and agencies off campus (e.g., families, medical providers, counselors, religious groups, non-profit organizations, etc.) and on campus. In IHE, the focus of this book, everyone, including faculty, staff, and students, plays a role in developing a warm campus. Such supportive communities exist when "members look out for one another, value the individual, promote a collective identity, and are not afraid to speak out when they recognize distress" (Bertram, 2010, pp. 31–32). This environment cannot exist if mental health disorders continue to be stigmatized. Anti-stigma, or stigma reduction, programs are essential as IHE move forward. Stigma reduction initiatives can include shifting to asset-oriented language use on campus, making mental health services accessible, and correcting stereotypes and misconceptions (Condra et al., 2015; Davey, 2013; Pedersen & Paves, 2014; Tucker et al., 2013; Wood, 2012).

Service provision must be actualized in ways that are humanizing and maintain students' privacy. This could include communicating clear policies (e.g., confidentiality commitments and release authorizations), locating offices in convenient and private settings, and creating supportive cultures. Supportive cultures can grow by improving and increasing mental health literacy (DiPlacito-DeRango, 2016; Murphy & Baines, 2015; Tucker et al., 2013). In these ways, campuses move to normalize mental health disorders and encourage students to access the services available to them. The following section addresses mental health awareness and knowledge of both students and faculty.

Promoting Awareness and Increasing Knowledge of Mental Health

Students With and Without Mental Health Disorders Lack Information

Research indicates that many college students with mental health disorders lack the knowledge to effectively manage their disability. One major barrier is being unaware of their rights and responsibilities as a college/university student with a disability (Condra et al., 2015). Title II of the Americans with Disabilities Act (ADA) and Section 504 of the Rehabilitation Act or 1973 (Section 504) prohibit discrimination on the basis of disability. These laws protect all individuals with disabilities, including students in elementary, secondary, and postsecondary settings. In IHE, Section 504 entitles eligible students to appropriate academic adjustments. "Academic adjustments may include auxiliary aids and services, as well as modifications to academic requirements as necessary to ensure equal educational opportunity (USDOE, 2011). Such academic adjustments can be gained if the student with the disability reports (provides documentation) that he/she has a disability to the appropriate office on campus and requests services. It is the responsibility of the college student to self-disclose and obtain academic adjustments, if needed. Students who are unaware of their rights and responsibilities are not likely to secure the supports to which they are legally entitled.

Those who are aware of their rights and responsibilities must also know how to access services on campus. Unfortunately, many college students with disabilities are either unaware of the services available to them, do not know where to go for help, or do not know the process for accessing services (Condra et al., 2015; Oswalt & Riddock, 2007; Pedersen & Paves, 2014; Quinn et al., 2009). These barriers are exacerbated by offices of student support services that are located in areas of campus either not known to or not readily accessible to students with disabilities (DiPlacito-DeRango, 2016; Quinn et al., 2009; Silverman, 2008). IHE can do a better job of educating students with mental health disorders about available services on campus and make these services readily available. Additionally, IHE can help students become self-determined human beings. "Professionals can do much to advocate for and support students, but ultimately students must learn to advocate for themselves and support each other" (Bertram, 2010, p. 32).

Students currently without mental health disorders also lack mental health knowledge. As a result, social stigma may exist. In this space, stereotypes and misinformation can breed fear and discrimination, which is detrimental for students with mental illness. Lack of knowledge also impedes the ability of college students without mental illness to help peers in crisis. If one cannot spot indicators of mental distress or is unaware of the services available on campus, he/she cannot intervene in positive ways. Bystander training has recently been encouraged to address this (Bertram, 2010; Prince, 2015; Wood, 2012). As Bertram (2010) asserts, "distressed students are more likely to go to their peers with their problems. Thus, it is critical that students are offered this information in a format that will give them agency when a friend is in need" (p. 31). Moreover, lacking mental health literacy can be personally harmful. Just because a student is currently mentally healthy, that does not mean he/she will never experience mental distress. Enhancing mental health awareness and knowledge for all college students is beneficial.

Faculty and Staff Lack Information

Research also indicates that many college faculty and staff lack awareness and knowledge of mental health issues on campus. They may lack knowledge of students' rights (Condra, et al., 2015). Consequently, some faculty and staff do not realize their legal obligation to make academic adjustments. They may be uninformed about the services to which they could refer students or the process to do so (Condra et al., 2015; Mitchell et al., 2012; Storrie, Ahern, & Tuckett, 2012) and unaware of the importance of referring students for non-acute, non-crisis mental health matters (Mitchell et al., 2012). Therefore, they are not able to advise students properly. Also, they may lack awareness of particular mental health issues, early warning signs of mental illness, and how such disorders manifest for individual students (Storrie et al., 2012; Tinklin et al., 2005). As such, they are unable to identify and intervene in a timely manner for students who are at-risk.

Additionally, some faculty and staff may be unsure of how to make appropriate academic adjustments in their courses (Condra, et al., 2015; Tinklin et al., 2005). A lack of effective accommodations can negatively affect the learning environment. In some cases reluctance to make academic adjustments is related to faculty and staff holding negative attitudes about individuals with mental illness (questioning their capacity to succeed) or the concern that making accommodations will diminish academic standards and compromise the rigor of the program (Condra et al., 2015). Such misunderstandings or misperceptions can contribute to a "knowledge gap" (Storrie et al., 2012, p. 101) where faculty and staff are unsure of or ill-prepared to fulfill their role as a "first-line responder" (DiPlacito-DeRango, 2016, p. 7) and college/ university students with mental health issues do not receive the academic or psychological support to which they are entitled. Training and awareness campaigns can mitigate this knowledge gap, not only for faculty and staff but also for college/university students.

Campus Training and Awareness Campaigns

Numerous researchers (Asidao & Sevig, 2014; Bertram, 2010; DiPlacito-DeRango, 2016; Hunt & Eisenberg, 2010; Mitchell et al., 2012) discuss the importance of "gatekeeper" training. As defined by the U.S. Surgeon General (USDHHS, 2012), gatekeepers are community members:

Who have face-to-face contact with large numbers of community members as part of their usual routine. They may be trained to identify personas at risk of suicide and refer them to treatment or supporting services as appropriate. Examples include clergy, first responders, pharmacists, caregivers, and those employed in institutional settings, such as schools, prisons, and the military. (p. 139)

By extending this definition beyond the P-12 setting to the college/university environment, faculty and staff in IHE can be considered gatekeepers. Gatekeeper training aims to educate individuals on identifying and referring students who may benefit from mental health services. This model is preventive in nature. It attempts to provide faculty and staff with the knowledge and skills to make early referrals. In turn, this should increase the number of students attaining mental health services before their situations escalate to acute mental distress and reduce the number of students who commit suicide.

One example of gatekeeper training is Question, Persuade, and Refer (QPR). QPR is nationally recognized and empirically based. It involves teaching:

Front-line people (e.g., faculty, staff, friends) how to recognize the warning signs of suicide, including verbal, behaviors, and situational clues, and provides guidelines on how to question persons about suicidal thoughts, persuade them to get help and refer them for help. (Asidao & Sevig, 2014, p. 136)

It is based on the notion that early recognition and early intervention are critical. Like Cardiopulmonary Resuscitation (CPR), it is an intervention "designed to increase the chance of survival in the event of a crisis" (What is QPR?). Another example of gatekeeper training is Campus Connect. It is "experientially based and teaches constituents to recognize distress and mental health issues in students, use basic helping techniques, and refer others to resources that could provide help" (Bertram, 2010, p. 31). In addition to providing information, Campus Connect uses multiple exercises and role play activities to increase communication skills, particularly empathic listening skills, of trainees. This evidence-based model builds on connectedness and uses culturally appropriate approaches. Both trainings are similar in that they promote community engagement and comprehensive strategies to save college/university students' lives. For more information on QPR or Campus Connect, please visit their websites.

Though useful, trainings like QPR and Campus Connect are not the only options for increasing awareness of mental health disorders. Training can be targeted to particular members of the campus community, and it can be provided via multiple avenues. Training for faculty and staff, who interact with college/university students on a weekly, if not daily, basis should incorporate wide-ranging information. This includes information about prevalent mental health disorders (particularly, characteristics and evidence-based academic interventions), the process students use to obtain accommodations, supporting students by using existing campus resources, and complying with confidentiality policies (Condra et al., 2015). Academic advisors, in particular, may benefit from such training (Wood, 2012). They have an opportunity to get to know their advisees as a "whole person." Academically, advisors have access to mid-term grades, course schedules, and transcripts, which enable them to see how the student is doing across all courses. Typically, advisors also have designated advising times where they meet individually with advisees and check-in on their overall well-being and adjustment to college/university. That is not to say these conversations do not or cannot occur organically with course faculty. In many cases the time and space for such conversations is intentionally built in to the formal academic advising structure (though it may not always be capitalized on).

Training to increase mental health literacy can be provided in multiple ways. It can occur at orientation for new faculty and staff and through new or enhanced existing professional development for current faculty and staff (DiPlacito-DeRango, 2016). Though initial trainings are important, one-shot deals are not enough. Training should be ongoing (Barr, 2014). Campus Counseling Centers often play a role in such professional development but are not solely responsible. Web-based self-training modules exist and centers for teaching and learning can host workshops, professional learning communities, and conferences on mental health (DiPlacito-DeRango, 2016). Combined, these approaches provide faculty and staff myriad opportunities to engage in meaningful conversations about mental health. In this way, information is made accessible in multiple formats. That is not to say that mere exposure to information will positively affect dispositions and behaviors. Admittedly, some employees could simply comply, complete training sessions, then not examine and/or change their role in promoting mental well-being on campus. For any training to work, the learner must authentically want to gain new understandings and use this new knowledge to change something for the better. While training focuses more on the individual or particular groups, general awareness campaigns have the potential to reach the masses.

Public information campaigns can increase awareness and work to reduce the stigma of mental illness on campus. Such campaigns can share statistics about mental health issues and provide mental health resources (Pedersen & Paves, 2014; Price, 2015). They not only benefit faculty and staff but also students with and without mental health disorders, especially when intentionally planned and implemented. Publications, forums, and tabling events are typical approaches to advertising services (Asidao & Sevig, 2014; DiPlacito-DeRango, 2016; Murphy & Baines, 2015). Such strategies reach a limited pool of students. Attention needs to be paid to all members of the campus community, including graduate students, commuter students, and online students. Due to their specialized study located in an isolated part of campus or their primary residence off campus, these students may not see traditional marketing campaigns (Oswalt & Riddock, 2007). To reach the broadest audience, additional tools like websites, online modules, and mobile phone apps can be used to disseminate information and provide services to support mental health (DiPlacito-DeRango, 2016; Murphy & Baines, 2015).

Many members of the campus community (students, faculty, and staff) have poor mental health literacy. As a result, students are not likely to pursue services and faculty and staff are less prepared to make student referrals for services. If an overarching goal for IHE is to positively affect mental health, or flourishing, then campuses should create cultures that cultivate acceptance and awareness. Increased mental health literacy is an important part of the solution. Yet knowledge alone is not enough to reduce the number of acute mental health crises on campus. Knowledge should be accompanied by action.

Applying Newly Acquired Knowledge of Mental Health Issues

There are multiple ways IHE faculty and staff can apply what they have learned about mental health in small-group and large-group settings. Such interventions range on a continuum from low-intensity to high-intensity and can be implemented by a single faculty member or a group of specialized staff. In the following section, I will discuss curriculum adjustments, face-to-face interventions, and online interventions that are associated with college/university student mental health. These strategies can be applied by faculty and staff in all academic programs across campus.

Engaged Learning

Civic engagement, as mentioned previously, is a predictor of college student mental health (Fink, 2014). Higher levels of civic engagement are associated with flourishing. Across campus, such engagement can be promoted through Living-Learning Programs (LLPs). As defined in the *National Study of Living-Learning Programs* report, LLPs are "programs that involve undergraduate students who live together in a discrete portion of a residence hall (or the entire hall) and participate in academic and/or extra-curricular programming designed especially for them" (Inkelas, Brower, Crawford, Hummel, Pope, & Zeller, 2004, p. I-1). In these settings, students have opportunities to regularly collaborate with peers, faculty, and community members on specialized projects. Each LLP is designed around a common theme and typically includes community engagement. In addition to campus-wide initiatives like LLPs, civic engagement can be fostered in individual courses.

In the college classroom, engaged learning has been associated with student mental health and well-being (Swaner, 2007). The concept of engaged learning is often used in two distinct, though not entirely separate, ways. First, it draws from experiential learning theory, where the individual interacts with the environment and actively co-constructs shared meaning. In this way, the individual is actively involved in or "engaged" in his/her learning (Swaner, 2007). Second, it is associated with civic engagement, where students participate or are "engaged" with communities. Such engagement occurs on multiple levels, including local, regional, national, international, and global spheres. It has mutual benefits for private life and public life, both preparing students for citizenship in a participatory democracy and enhancing the community (Swaner, 2007). Common models of engaged learning include service learning, community-based research, collaborative learning, and problem-based learning (Swaner, 2007). Internships and interdisciplinary co-teaching are other examples. That is not to say, however, that these approaches are prevalent in IHEs. Although research indicates that many of the aforementioned engaged learning pedagogies "enhance learning, increase content mastery, encourage critical thinking, and foster personal development," such learning opportunities are "offered only on a limited and elective basis on most campuses" (Swaner, 2007, p. 20). Engaged learning could be promoted by both departments within Student Affairs and throughout academic departments. At the instructor-level, additional curricular adjustments can be made to enhance and support student mental health.

Curriculum Infusion

In addition to adopting a particular pedagogical framework, faculty can promote college student well-being by infusing aspects of mental health into the curriculum. Here, I borrow Mitchell et al.'s (2012) definition of curriculum infusion: "developing class activities and assignments that introduce faculty and students to mental health topics such as depression, anxiety, eating disorders, or suicide while at the same time focusing on academic content" (p. 25). Major assignments can be scaffolded around mental health literacy and texts about mental health issues can be assigned as required readings (DiPlacito-DeRango, 2016; Savini, 2016). Not all faculty and staff are knowledgeable in this area, so collaboration with qualified personnel is important during all aspects of course design and delivery.

Such curriculum infusion can be thoughtfully merged within numerous relevant disciplines. One university, for example, established partnerships between its Mental Health Awareness Committee and faculty in various academic programs to embed mental health literacy into particular courses. Here, a Visual Studies program used art exhibits to raise awareness about emotional distress, emotional wellness, and resiliency. The Design for New Media class created posters and Public Service Announcements to increase awareness about mental health issues and related campus resources. The Applied Marking Techniques class developed a marketing campaign on behalf of Counseling Services (Mitchell et al., 2012). In each of these cases, topics related to mental health were incorporated to help students achieve course objectives. The study of mental health was not simply a course add-on. Rather, that topic served as a vehicle through which students learned course content and provided service to the campus community through such applied projects. As compared to traditional training programs, curriculum infusion produced more faculty interest and involvement in mental health promotion (Mitchell et al., 2012). Faculty awareness and action is essential in promoting well-being and in deterring mental health crises.

Faculty can take additional steps to increase mental health literacy in their own courses. They can build-in class time to announce mental health campus-wide events, distribute counseling center information, host speakers on mental health related topics, and include a statement about mental health in their syllabi (DiPlacito-DeRango, 2016; Mitchell et al., 2012; Savini, 2016). Referring to a previous point, faculty can create communities of learners. They can do this by lecturing less and integrating more collaborative projects.

They can also promote forums where students talk with each other to reduce isolation, in a way creating support groups (Quinn et al., 2009; Savini, 2016). Such forums could exist in face-to-face courses, online courses, and go beyond the classroom. One university even has a "buddying system" where second-year and first-year students are paired; the returning student offering support to the new student until he/she is acclimated to college life (Quinn et al., 2009). Additionally, faculty can intervene early. Surveying the class, checking-in with individual students, and referring students appropriately are effective strategies to address mental distress (Mitchell et al., 2012; Savini, 2016). Early intervention is more likely to occur when faculty have received training and taken the time to get to know their students. All of these examples demonstrate ways faculty can make adjustments in the classroom to better support student well-being. Beyond curriculum infusion, entire courses can be offered to address mental health issues.

General Course Offerings

Research indicates that general course offerings can be effective in promoting and facilitating mental health on campus. Such courses can disseminate information on campus mental health resources and help students better understand themselves as developing social and emotional beings (Conley, Durlak, & Dickson, 2013; Wood, 2012). Courses can also help students develop generalizable life skills that allow them to face the challenges and stress of college life and learning (Hartley, 2012; Silverman, 2008). These life skills can include, but are not limited to, time management, study skills and habits, self-care, and relaxation (Damer & Melendres, 2011; Hartley, 2012). Such skills can be connected to resilience, "the process of, capacity for, or outcome of successful adaptation despite challenging or threatening circumstance," and protective factors, "the qualities of persons or contexts that predict positive outcomes under high-risk conditions" (Hartley, 2012, p. 38). Resilience and protective factors are positively associated with mental health. Programs that focus on building resilience through skills-oriented approaches are associated with increased self-esteem, self-perception, self-confidence, self-leadership, and prosocial behaviors and related to decreased emotional distress, specifically depression, anxiety, and stress (Conley, Durlak, & Dickson, 2013; Hartley, 2012). Such courses enhance social and emotional development by teaching life skills that will help students be successful in academic and non-academic settings. To be constructive, programming should be both intentionally designed and delivered.

IHE have approached general course offerings to promote mental health in several ways. For instance, a medical school offers a one-semester course entitled "Mind–Body Medicine: an Experiential Elective." The 10-week course meets weekly for two-hour sessions. Students who volunteer to participate are first led through a didactic presentation, covering topics related to physiological responses to stress and ways to cope with stress. Small groups of students are then given the opportunity to practice specific skills related to the concept of the week. Additionally, students are expected to complete homework (physical activity and meditation). Results indicate that this mind-body course reduced participants' anxiety levels as students used newly developed skills "to cope more effectively with the stresses of medical school" (Finkelstein, Brownstein, Scott, & Lan, 2007, pp. 262-263).

As another example, a university offers a two-semester course to undergraduate students entitled "Risk and Resilience (R&R) in Urban Teens," which focuses on "mental health promotion, stress reduction, and resilience" (Shatkin et al., 2016, p. 205). Semester One, structured didactically, provides students with theories and practices about stress, stress reduction, and resilience. Semester Two, organized as a service-learning project, provides students the opportunity to apply their newly acquired knowledge by teaching skills and techniques intended to reduce stress to local high school students. Results indicate that, compared to controls, R&R students self-reported improvement in their mental health. "Specifically, they reported less perceived stress, better coping skills, and a reduction in dysfunctional attitudes" (Shatkin et al., 2016, p. 207).

At another IHE, a seminar on psychological wellness was offered to first-year undergraduate students. The seminar occurred weekly for 50 minutes during the fall and spring semesters. It covered a range of topics associated with psychosocial adjustment and stress management. Each seminar contained four elements: didactic instruction, journal writing about experiences and reactions, participation in class activities, and skills practice homework. Results indicate that students benefitted by an increased sense of well-being and by better managing college-related stress (Conley, Travers, & Bryant, 2013). Furthermore, the authors claim that such a course, "by taking a universal approach… can be applied to—or customized for—different campuses, contexts, and special populations" (Conley, Travers, & Bryant, 2013, p. 84). In other words, this model can be replicated throughout IHE and tailored to meet the needs of specific colleges/universities.

Admittedly, there are numerous ways to structure courses for mental health promotion. Such courses vary in size, interventions used, duration, audience, and format (Conley, Durlak, & Dickson, 2013). Taken together, the examples of skills-based courses presented here suggest that the explicit teaching of skills to enhance resilience and build protective factors are effective in enhancing mental health. Courses ranging from one semester to two semesters have been found to reduce stress and anxiety while increasing personal resources to successfully cope with college challenges. Common to the examples included here is an emphasis on both theory and practice. Students were provided conceptual schemes and evidence-based interventions and required to use their newly developed skills. Moreover, students were actively engaged in multiple settings–inside the classroom and outside the classroom (or as some students refer to it, "real life"). This suggests that one's mental status is not necessarily pre-determined or fixed. Students can learn factors that enhance mental health, hone coping skills, and implement effective practices. In this way, students act as agents to positively affect their own well-being.

Additionally, general course offerings could be tailored to two primary populations: new students and returning students. If early intervention is effective in mediating mental health crises, then it stands to reason that programming should be provided as soon as students first arrive on campus, even during orientation. But programming should not stop there. Although one- or two-semester courses have been found effective in helping students learn and apply stress coping interventions presently, some research indicates that they do not necessarily have long-term effects beyond the intervention period (Conley, Travers, & Bryant, 2013; Shatkin et al., 2016). This suggests that one-shot course offerings may need boosters, follow-up seminars, to have enduring usefulness. Furthermore, the models discussed here were offered to students on a volunteer basis. To reach a broader audience, IHE may include similar courses as part of the required coursework for all majors. In this way, such proactive and preventive interventions become "systemic in higher education" as they are "integrated into the routine structure and programming of higher education institutions" (Conley, Durlak, & Dickson, 2013, p. 297).

Mindfulness Training

In addition to skills-based interventions, mindfulness-based interventions have been found effective in promoting mental well-being. Here, I use mindfulness to mean "the awareness that emerges through purposefully paying nonjudgmental attention to present moment experiences" (Bergen-Cico, Possemato, & Cheon, 2013, p. 349). One example of such training is Mindfulness-Based Stress Reduction (MBSR). Students participate in discussions about meta-cognition and the mind–body–psychological connection; they also practice multiple types of meditation and guided body scan (Bergen-Cico et al., 2013). Upon completion of this training, students reported significant levels of improvement in mindfulness and self-compassion, two measures of psychological health. Likewise, a Mindfulness-Based Stress Management (MBSM/Mindful-Gym) program produced positive results regarding mental health. Training included didactic and experiential methods which were "designed for students to pay attention to the present moment, relaxing moments, and grateful moments in life" (Phang, Mukhtar, Ibrahim, Keng, & Sidik, 2015, p. 1118). Results indicate that students benefitted from reduced perceived stress and mental distress and increased mindfulness and self-efficacy. In a modified MBSR program, participants were provided information on coping strategies during group sessions and practiced new techniques on their own at home. Results reveal that students receiving MBSR training "increased their use of problem-focused coping," and those students with self-reported "high scores on neuroticism benefitted from the intervention in terms of reduced avoidance-focused coping and an increase in seeking social support" (Halland, deVibe, Solhaug, Friborg, Rosenvinge, Tyssen, Sorlie, & Bjorndal, 2015, p. 388). Each of these measures is associated with mental health.

Mindfulness training can be used in conjunction with general course offerings and/or embedded in courses to promote college/university student mental health. Both are similar in that they incorporate theory and practice, and they have relatively immediate results with positive outcomes reported within weeks or months of intervention initiation. They differ, though, in their duration. While courses can last a semester or two, mindfulness trainings typically last five to 10 weeks. Because mindfulness training is delivered in small groups, over short periods of time, without the expectation of students to disclose personal information, it can be "a relatively cost-, time- and labour-effective intervention" (Phang et al., 2015, p. 1128).

Online Interventions

Thus far, discussion has focused on campus-based interventions, as in those courses or seminars delivered by faculty and staff in a face-to-face format.

This delivery method pertains to "traditional" college students and overlooks "online" students. As our society continues to embrace technology, the number of "distance learners" will likely grow. Students taking mostly online courses may benefit from a different approach to mental health promotion.

Technology has been found effective in promoting mental health awareness and as a vehicle for intervention (Asidao & Sevig, 2014; Barr, 2014; Hintz, Frazier, & Meredith, 2015; Koydemir & Sun-Selisik, 2016; Wood, 2012). IHE websites can serve as repositories of information on mental health education and available campus and electronic services. MiTalk is one such example. It is an "interactive, multimedia Web site" that provides students "with knowledge and skills to get help or to help friends who may be in distress because of depression, anxiety, social identity, trauma, stress management, or other mental health concerns" (Asidao & Sevig, 2014, p. 137). YouTube and Facebook can also be used for mental health outreach (Asidao & Sevig, 2014).

In addition, technology can support student development through online workshops. Though composition may differ slightly, web-based interventions "often contain psychoeducation delivered via text, video or audio, assignments, and personalized feedback" (Hintz et al., 2015, p. 138). One university offered a 4-module training via Google sites focused on common college stressors and past, present, future control theory. Each module consisted of a narrated presentation, student examples, and application exercises. Upon workshop completion, participants who practiced present control reported less perceived stress and reductions in anxiety and depression (Hintz et al., 2015). As another example, an 8-week online intervention focusing on strengths and goals, emotion regulation, pro-social skills, problem-solving and decision-making skills, and motivation was offered to first-year students at another university. Participants who completed the 5-module training (including both didactic and experiential components) reported improved well-being in several areas, "namely subjective happiness, life satisfaction, subjective happiness, ontological well-being and psychological well-being" (Koydemir & Sun-Selisik, 2016, p. 440). This suggests that "well-being promotion through technology can be effective in facilitating a flourishing life among students" (Koydemir & Sun-Selisik, 2016, p. 442). Though only two studies are presented here, these results support similar research in the field.

There are many benefits to online mental health resources. They have the potential to reach a large audience, regardless of students' proximity to the college/university, and can be sustained (Barr, 2014; Hintz et al., 2015; Koydemir & Sun-Selisik, 2016). Electronic resources may be more readily accessed by students due to their convenience as they can be used at times that fit students' schedules and allow for user anonymity (Hintz et al., 2015; Wood, 2012). Yet, given that some students are not digital natives or do not have access to adequate technology, digital approaches should not be the only way to enhance mental well-being. IHE should use a multifaceted approach that is inclusive of the diverse student body.

Campus Mental Health Policies

Without a common mission and cohesive procedures, mental health promotion initiatives will likely be sporadic and disjointed. If communicated superficially or to certain individuals (Student Affairs staff rather than Academic Affairs faculty, for example), then useful policy will not be systemic. Rather, it will be implemented in pockets across campus. Such random practices are potentially harmful as they allow students to slip through the cracks. Unfortunately, this is often the case. "Institutionalized, coordinated, and sustainable mental health policies have yet to emerge in post-secondary schools" (DiPlacito-DeRango, 2016, p. 3). Such underdeveloped policies are seen as a barrier to college/university student mental well-being, and as such, a place for reform (Condra et al., 2015; DiPlacito-DeRango, 2016; Murphy & Baines, 2015; Silverman, 2008; Wood, 2012). A unified and comprehensive approach to mental health is desired.

Campus-wide policies should be thorough and clear. They can include guidelines for promoting mental well-being in a preventive manner and specific procedures for responding during mental health crises. Such "student-friendly policies" are seen as proactive, not punitive (Murphy & Baines, 2015, p. 23). It should be clear how the campus will establish policy and review policy. Policy should be regularly evaluated for relevance to the overall mission of the college/university, current application, and usefulness (Condra et al., 2015; DiPlacito-DeRango, 2016; Murphy & Baines, 2015; Wood, 2012). Furthermore, policy should be shared with everyone who is responsible for implementing it. Both the "how to" (detailing steps) and the "why to" (garnering buy-in) should be communicated. A policy on paper and not enacted is ineffective. It is recommended that a multi-disciplinary committee convene to create such policy.

Many IHE now have committees of administrators, faculty, and staff who collaborate to establish and review mental health policy. Though common in IHE, these committees may differ organizationally and operationally. For example, such committees go by various names, including the Campus

Assessment Team, the Student Behavior Consultation Team, the Assessment and Care Team, the Student of Concern Committee, and many others (Eells & Rockland-Miller, 2011; Prince, 2015). Their mission and purpose also vary. Committees can be divided into three categories: those that focus on student behavior assessment and intervention; those that primarily manage crises; and those that combine both approaches (Eells & Rockland-Miller, 2011). In addition to setting campus-wide policy, these teams can meet to evaluate individual student cases. Through early intervention, such teams review students "who demonstrate behaviors that are disruptive or worrisome," and provide support before problems escalate (Prince, 2015, p. 7). They also engage in a process of "threat assessment," where team members determine if a specific student poses foreseeable danger to him-/her-self or others and decide on steps to address the threat (Bishop, 2010; Eells & Rockland-Miller, 2011).

Committees are unique in other ways. Team responsibilities and composition differ. For example, teams may set policy, communicate policy, manage student cases, foster cross-campus collaborations with other groups promoting wellness, and/or train and support academic departments (Eells & Rockland-Miller, 2011; Murphy & Baines, 2015). Membership may include representatives from counseling services, student discipline office, campus safety, health services, academic affairs, student disabilities office, legal counsel, athletics, Greek life, and/or faculty (DiPlacito-DeRango, 2016; Eells & Rockland-Miller, 2011). Teams have case review procedures, documentation procedures, and referral sources, yet these factors may be actualized differently from IHE to IHE (Eells & Rockland-Miller, 2011). Regardless of these differences, all teams share the common goal of promoting mental health on their campus. This goal remains important as the prevalence of mental illness in college/university continues to rise. Policy-setting and -enforcing committees are important in addressing this issue as they "provide a venue for making caring, well-reasoned, and appropriate decisions about students" who may be in experiencing mental distress (Eells & Rockland-Miller, 2011, p. 22).

Yet campuses are not alone in this endeavor. Numerous mental health resources in the local and broader communities exist. IHE can work with these agencies to enhance mental health promotion on campus. National organizations and commercial services, such as the following, can be of use: The JED Foundation (Barr, 2014; Hoover, 2003; Silverman, 2008; Wood, 2012); Campusblues.com (Hoover, 2003); Active Minds on Campus (Hoover, 2003); Center for the Study of College Student Health (Wood, 2012); Mentality

(Wood, 2012); The Mental Health and Wellness Association (Wood, 2012); The Suicide Prevention Resource Center (Silverman, 2008); The American Association of Suicidology (Silverman, 2008); The Garret Lee Smith Memorial Act (Silverman, 2008); and The Historically Black Colleges and Universities National Resource Center (Silverman, 2008). The aforementioned agencies serve as examples and do not constitute a comprehensive list. They are meant to be used as potential resources, starting points, for IHE looking to strengthen mental health policies on campus.

CONCLUSION

If flourishing, as Keyes (2005 & 2007) presents it, leads to a good life, then IHE ultimately should provide students the knowledge, skills, and opportunities to flourish. This occurs not only in the absence of mental illness but with numerous factors associated with mental health, not the least of which are self-knowledge, a sense of belonging, and engagement. Today, the prevalence of mental illness on college/universities campuses is growing. Such mental health challenges prevent college/university students from flourishing. Wait-to-fail models where mental health services are provide after a serious event occurs are antiquated. They neither support the student in crisis nor the campus community. Current scholars in the field call for new initiatives, initiatives that promote mental well-being and prevent mental distress on a systemic level (Bertram, 2010; Conley, Durlak, & Dickson, 2013; Hartley, 2012; Hunt & Eisenberg, 2010; Murphy & Baines, 2015; Swaner, 2007; Wood, 2012). The responsibility for creating campuses where students can flourish is no longer the sole domain of counseling centers or student health services. This requires comprehensive, integrated policies and the collaboration of all stakeholders.

This chapter focused on strategies for college/university faculty and staff who do not have extensive knowledge or experience in fields related to mental health. It described several best practices, such as building community, gaining mental health literacy, and adjusting academic curriculum that are effective in promoting mental health. These initiatives can be instituted throughout and across departments with relative ease. Often, such initiatives do not require large amounts of money, time, or effort. They do, however, require support from all campus members. "Effective and creative intervention [is] imperative" (Bertram, 2010, p. 33). Students are best served by a "multidimensional approach that combines short-term therapeutic services with educational outreach, community support, and infrastructure for student empowerment"

(Bertram, 2010, p. 33). In this way, "the campus is not made a treatment facility, but instead offers the tools for students to understand and negotiate the emotional, psychological, and intellectual components of these issues" (Bertram, 2010, p. 33). A concerted and effort and innovative approach to mental well-being is essential as IHE move forward.

REFERENCES

Asidao, C., & Sevig, T. (2014). Reaching in to reach out: One counseling centers journey in developing a new outreach approach. *Journal of College Student Psychotherapy, 28*(2), 132–143. doi:10.1080/87568225.2014.883881

Barr, B. (2014). Identifying and addressing the mental health needs of online students in higher education. *Online Journal of Distance Learning Administration, 17*(2).

Bergen-Cico, D., Possemato, K., & Cheon, S. (2013). Examining the efficacy of a brief mindfulness based stress reduction (Brief MBSR) program on psychological health. *Journal of American College Health, 61*(6), 348–360. doi:10.1080/07448481.2013.813853 PMID:23930749

Bertram, M. (2010). Student mental health: Reframing the problem.. *About Campus: Enriching the Student Learning Experience, 15*(4), 30–32. doi:10.1002/abc.20033

Bishop, J. B. (2010). The counseling center: An undervalued resource in recruitment, retention, and risk management. *Journal of College Student Psychotherapy, 24*(4), 248–260. doi:10.1080/87568225.2010.509219

Condra, M., Dineen, M., Gills, H., Jack-Davies, A., & Condra, E. (2015). Academic accommodations for postsecondary students with mental health disabilities in Ontario, Canada: A review of the literature and reflections on emerging issues. *Journal of Postsecondary Education and Disability, 28*(3), 277–291.

Conley, C. S., Durlak, J. A., & Dickson, D. A. (2013). An evaluative review of outcome research on universal mental health promotion and prevention programs for higher education students. *Journal of American College Health, 61*(5), 286–301. doi:10.1080/07448481.2013.802237 PMID:23768226

Conley, C. S., Travers, L. V., & Bryant, F. B. (2013). Promoting psychosocial adjustment and stress management in first-year college students: The benefits of engagement in psychosocial wellness seminar. *Journal of American College Health, 61*(2), 75–86. doi:10.1080/07448481.2012.754757 PMID:23409857

Damer, D. E., & Melendres, L. T. (2011). Tackling Test Anxiety: A group for college students. *Journal for Specialists in Group Work, 36*(3), 163–177. doi:10.1080/01933922.2011.586016

Davey, G. C. L. (2013). Mental health & stigma. *Psychology Today*. Retrieved from https://www.psychologytoday.com/blog/why-we-worry/201308/mental-health-stigma

DiPlacito-DeRango, M. L. (2016). Acknowledge the barriers to better the practices: support for student mental health in higher education. *The Canadian Journal for the Scholarship of Teaching and Learning, 7*(2).

Eells, G. T., & Rockland-Miller, H. S. (2011). Assessing and responding to disturbed and disturbing students: Understanding the role of administrative teams in institutions of higher education. *Journal of College Student Psychotherapy, 25*(1), 8–23. doi:10.1080/87568225.2011.532470

Fink, J. E. (2014). Flourishing: Exploring predictors of mental health within the college environment. *Journal of American College Health, 62*(6), 380–388. doi:10.1080/07448481.2014.917647 PMID:24779485

Finkelstein, C., Brownstein, A., Scott, C., & Lan, Y. (2007). Anxiety and stress reduction in medical education: An intervention. *Medical Education, 41*(3), 258–264. doi:10.1111/j.1365-2929.2007.02685.x PMID:17316210

Halland, E., deVibe, M., Solhaug, I., Friborg, O., Rosenvinge, J. H., Tyssen, R., & Bjorndal, A. et al. (2015). Mindfulness training improves problem-focused coping in psychology and medical students: Results from a randomized controlled trial. *College Student Journal, 49*(3), 387–398.

Hartley, M. T. (2012). Assessing and promoting resilience: An additional tool to address the increasing number of college students with psychological problems. *Journal of College Counseling, 15*(1), 37–51. doi:10.1002/j.2161-1882.2012.00004.x

Hoover, E. (2003). More help for troubled students. *The Chronicle of Higher Education, 50*(15), A25–A26.

Hunt, J., & Eisenberg, D. (2010). Mental health problems and help-seeking behavior among college students. *The Journal of Adolescent Health*, *46*(1), 3–10. doi:10.1016/j.jadohealth.2009.08.008 PMID:20123251

Inkelas, K. K., Brower, A. M., Crawford, S., Hummel, M., Pope, D., & Zeller, W. J. (2004). *National study of living-learning programs*. Columbus, OH: Association of College & University Housing Officers International; Retrieved from http://www.ms07.umd.edu/Appendices/NationalLivingLearningStudy.pdf

JED. (2016). *What we do*. Retrieved from https://www.jedfoundation.org/what-we-do/

Keyes, C. L. M. (2005). Mental illness and/or mental health? Investigating axioms of the complete state model of health. *Journal of Counseling and Clinical Psychology*, *73*(3), 539–548. doi:10.1037/0022-006X.73.3.539 PMID:15982151

Keyes, C. L. M. (2007). Promoting and protecting mental health as flourishing: A complementary strategy for improving national mental health. *The American Psychologist*, *62*(2), 95–108. doi:10.1037/0003-066X.62.2.95 PMID:17324035

Koydemir, S., & Sun-Selisik, Z. E. (2016). Well-being on campus: Testing the effectiveness of an online strengths-based intervention for first year college students. *British Journal of Guidance & Counselling*, *44*(4), 434–446. doi:10.1080/03069885.2015.1110562

Kraft, D. P. (2009). Mens sana: The growth of mental health in the American college health association. *Journal of American College Health*, *58*(3), 267–275. doi:10.1080/07448480903297546 PMID:19959441

Kraft, D. P. (2009). One hundred years of college mental health. *Journal of American College Health*, *59*(6), 477–481. doi:10.1080/07448481.2011.569964 PMID:21660801

Mitchell, S. L., Darrow, S. A., Haggerty, M., Neill, T., Carvalho, A., & Uschold, C. (2012). Curriculum infusion as college student mental health promotion strategy. *Journal of College Student Psychotherapy*, *26*(1), 22–38. doi:10.1080/87568225.2012.633038

Murphy, G., & Baines, J. (2015). Connecting the dots: Facilitating a positive university educational journey with an organisational mental health and wellbeing strategy. *Journal of the Australian & New Zealand Student Services Association, 46*(1), 20–27.

Oswalt, S. B., & Riddock, C. C. (2007). What to do about being overwhelmed: Graduate students, stress and university services. *The College of Student Affairs Journal, 27*(1), 24–44.

Pedersen, E. R., & Paves, A. P. (2014). Comparing perceived public stigma and personal stigma of mental health treatment seeking in a young adult sample. *Psychiatry Research, 219*(1), 143–150. doi:10.1016/j.psychres.2014.05.017 PMID:24889842

Phang, C. K., Mukhtar, F., Ibrahim, N., Keng, S., & Sidik, S. M. (2015). Effects of a brief mindfulness based intervention program for stress management among medical students: The Mindful-Gym randomized controlled study. *Advances in Health Science Education, 20*(5), 1115–1134. doi:10.1007/s10459-015-9591-3 PMID:25697124

Prince, J. P. (2015). University student counseling and mental health in the United States: Trends and challenges. *Mental Health & Prevention, 3*(1), 5–10. doi:10.1016/j.mhp.2015.03.001

Quinn, N., Wilson, A., MacIntyre, G., & Tinklin, T. (2009). People look at you differently: Students experience of mental health support within higher education. *British Journal of Guidance & Counselling, 37*(4), 405–418. doi:10.1080/03069880903161385

Savini, C. (2016). Are you being rigorous or just intolerant? How to promote mental health in the college classroom. *The Chronicle of Higher Education*. Retrieved from http://www.chronicle.com/article/Are-You-Being-Rigorous-or-Just/236341/

Shatkin, J. P., Diamond, U., Zhao, Y., DiMeglio, J., Chodaczek, M., & Bruzzese, J. M. (2016). Effects of a risk and resilience course on stress, coping skills, and cognitive strategies in college students. *Teaching of Psychology, 43*(3), 204–210. doi:10.1177/0098628316649457

Silverman, M. M. (2008). Campus security begins with caring. *The Chronicle of Higher Education, 54*(42), A51–A52.

Storrie, K., Ahern, K., & Tuckett, A. (2012). Crying in the halls: Supervising students with symptoms of emotional problems in the clinical practicum. *Teaching in Higher Education, 17*(1), 89–103. doi:10.1080/13562517.2011.590980

Swaner, L. E. (2007). Linking engaged learning, student mental health and well-being, and civic development: A review of the literature. *Liberal Education, 93*(1), 16–25.

Tinklin, T., Riddell, S., & Wilson, A. (2005). Support for students with mental health difficulties in higher education: The students perspective. *British Journal of Guidance & Counselling, 33*(4), 495–512. doi:10.1080/03069880500327496

Tucker, J. R., Hammer, J. H., Vogel, D. L., Bitman, R. L., Wade, N. G., & Maier, E. J. (2013). Disentangling self-stigma: Are mental illness and help-seeking self-stigmas different? *Journal of Counseling Psychology, 60*(4), 520–531. doi:10.1037/a0033555 PMID:23815629

U.S. Department of Education. (2011). *Students with disabilities preparing for postsecondary education: Know your rights and responsibilities.* Washington, DC: Office for Civil Rights. Retrieved from https://www2.ed.gov/about/offices/list/ocr/transition.html

U.S. Department of Health and Human Services (HHS) Office of the Surgeon General and National Action Alliance for Suicide Prevention. (2012). *National strategy for suicide prevention: Goals and objectives for action.* Washington, DC: HHS. Retrieved from https://www.surgeongeneral.gov/library/reports/national-strategy-suicide-prevention/full report.pdf

Wood, M. (2012). The state of mental health on college campuses. *Inquiry, 17*(1), 5–15.

Wrench, A., Garrett, R., & King, S. (2013). Guessing where the goal posts are: Managing health and well being during the transition to university studies. *Journal of Youth Studies, 16*(6), 730–746. doi:10.1080/13676261.2012.744814

Wrench, A., Garrett, R., & King, S. (2013). Guessing where the goal posts are: Managing health and well being during the transition to university studies. *Journal of Youth Studies, 16*(6), 730–746.

Chapter 6
What Is Next?
Future Considerations

Melissa Martin
State University of New York at Plattsburgh, USA

Jean Mockry
State University of New York at Plattsburgh, USA

Alison Puliatte
State University of New York at Plattsburgh, USA

Denise Simard
State University of New York at Plattsburgh, USA

Maureen E. Squires
State University of New York at Plattsburgh, USA

ABSTRACT

Because the possible problems related to mental health and well-being have been identified throughout the chapters of this book, the authors plan to implement and evaluate these strategies to help provide future directions and frameworks. This chapter describes a future research study and other explorations the authors wish to conduct. Specifically, the authors seek to measure preservice general and special educators' character dispositions (e.g., grit), and use these data to determine how to effectively help college students handle stress. Additionally, researchers hope to examine the use of technology in college classrooms to promote mindfulness. Finally, the implementation of strategies for the college classroom will be implemented and evaluated in teacher preparation coursework.

DOI: 10.4018/978-1-5225-3793-9.ch006

INTRODUCTION

As the authors of this book researched mental health on college campuses, a plethora of ideas about how to help students in coursework were posited. This section will explore some of these ideas.

OUR IMPLEMENTATION PLAN

Fink (2014) has identified potential strategies to promote well-being for college students through high-impact practices of learning and engagement. Fink (2014) indicates developing living-learning programs (LLPs) establishes socially supportive environments within campus residence halls. LLPs place a great deal of energy into building a sense of community within the dorms. These activities are vital for freshman transitioning to college, seeking a new social network. In our educator preparation program, we have seen the impact of building a sense of community. As we have developed and revised our programs, we have learned how essential it is for us to connect with our students immediately upon their arrival on campus and to connect to one another. Some strategies we implement include: using a cohort model for both faculty and students to progress through our 4- or 5-year programs; assigning the freshman instructor to each student as an academic advisor; looping with students for the freshman year; and incorporating community building activities and skill builders throughout the program. Each of these strategies allows teacher candidates to have a touch stone on campus within the first week of classes and helps build social and academic communities. In thinking about future considerations, we may want to research these strategies to determine if they do impact social well-being (regardless whether the student remains an education major or changes his or her major).

Social interactions and relationships and physical activity play vital roles maintaining positive mental health. The National Alliance on Mental Illness (NAMI) advocates college students build, "Connections with others, including involvement with campus and community activities, can help you protect your mental health. Explore opportunities through your campus student activities center and get involved in one or more of the following: Campus events; Campus clubs; Campus interest groups; Sports; Student organizations;

Volunteer activities" (p. 5). The authors would also advocate for more emphasis on programs to address improving social skills, communicating effectively, promoting positive coping skills, regulating emotions, fostering better self-care, developing sleep hygiene. Finally, we would support programs to offer parents strategies to facilitate their child's transition from high school to college. More specifically, strategies for offering emotional support and supporting college students to be resilient problem solvers.

In an effort to bring awareness and support to promoting positive mental health to the college campus, we are proposing, in collaboration of the Director of the Campus Psychological Center, to sponsor or mentor student led organizations, such as Active Minds, Inc. and JED. Active Minds is a national student led organization in which students plan and facilitate events on the college campus that focus on mental health awareness, education and advocacy. The purpose of supporting programs such as these is to remove the negative stigma around mental health and to create an environment of support and acceptance. Additionally, we have begun to collaborate with our colleagues in Student Affairs. With the support of campus leadership, we hope to participate in professional develop programs such as Mental Health First Aid.

Exploration of Technology for Support

The authors also want to explore the use of technology to support mental health in college. The use of apps or other online resources to de-escalate (from anxiety or stress) or participate in mindfulness activities will be examined. Specifically, does the use of these apps help students overcome some challenges or obstacles they may face in college and promote character dispositions (e.g., self-control, grit)?

During coursework, researchers plan to integrate mindfulness training and other interventions discussed in previous chapters to help students become gritty and to develop some of the other dispositional traits that can help with well-being. Moreover, instructors will integrate the use of technology to help facilitate some of the interventions.

In hopes of generalization and maintenance, the instructors will also discuss how students can use these tools when not in class. The goal of incorporating such strategies is for students to use them beyond the education coursework.

Specifically, we want students to explore a plethora of strategies (including technology) to gather an arsenal of possible ways to cope when faced with challenges in college. Some students may find one strategy is best for all types of challenges, while others may find a variety to be best. Regardless, we want our future teachers to be prepared, to have practiced strategies to cope, and to actually use these strategies during their teaching careers. To go full circle, we also want our students to teach their future students these skills when they become general or special education elementary teachers.

Future Research Study

The authors of this book also hope to examine the personality traits of current and future college students enrolled in a teacher preparation program at a university in upstate New York. Specifically, the we hope to explore the teacher traits (or personality traits) of future teachers while enrolled in college. These include grit, self-compassion, satisfaction with life, and perceived stress, among others. Additionally, scales examining emotional well-being, growth versus fixed mindsets, and mindfulness (e.g., Five Facet Mindfulness Questionnaire; see Baer, Smith, Hopkins, Krietemeyer, & Toney, 2006) will be administered.

Participants will include current and future students enrolled in a five-year teacher education program that will result in a bachelor's or master's' degree in childhood (elementary) and/or special education. Additionally, these participants will be enrolled at various stages of this program (e.g., freshman, sophomore, graduate) to examine if that may impact the magnitude and relationship of traits.

To examine these traits, researchers will administer various scales (e.g., 12 -item Grit Scale; see Duckworth, Peterson, Matthews, & Kelly, 2007). Relationships among the teacher trait variables and demographics will also be explored. Moreover, researchers hope to determine if a relationship exists among each trait. For example, is grit related to self-compassion for future educators?

Results of this study will help professors and instructors in college prepare coursework and/or needed interventions related to these traits (e.g., mindfulness training). Because, as we believe, the traits of teachers are important, it is essential to help college students develop and hone these skills before the first year of teaching.

ADDITIONAL GOALS

While the goal of this book was to develop a literature review about student well-being on college campuses and what instructors can do to prepare future teachers, we recognize additional research is needed. In the future, we hope to use the literature to build a theoretical framework to gain further knowledge about this problem. This will help provide additional future directions and help college instructors provide the needed tools for college students to combat stressors and develop the most essential character dispositions to become teachers. Moreover, we would like to explore how (or if) the well-being of college students, specifically in teacher education, impacts academic success and employment. While we can speculate and infer that these areas are impacted, it will be beneficial to investigate if our students have specific needs.

CONCLUSION

College can be difficult for some students. The stress of course requirements, new social settings, and employment may be overwhelming. Professors and instructors may need to (1) become knowledgeable about the mental health and well-being challenges on college campuses; (2) examine some reasons students may be successful (e.g., character dispositions) or unsuccessful (e.g., home life); and (3) explore possible strategies to implement in coursework and on campus. IHE can take meaningful actions to create environments in which college students flourish.

We encourage you all to examine these factors at your own institution and to implement effective strategies around campus and in your courses.

REFERENCES

Active Minds. (2017). *About us.* Retrieved April 11, 2017 from: http://www.activeminds.org/

Baer, R. A., Smith, G. T., Hopkins, J., Krietemeyer, J., & Toney, L. (2006). Using self-report assessment methods to explore facets of mindfulness. *Assessment, 13*(1), 27–45. doi:10.1177/1073191105283504 PMID:16443717

Duckworth, A. L., Peterson, C., Matthews, M. D., & Kelly, D. R. (2007). Grit: Perseverance and passion for long-term goals. *Journal of Personality and Social Psychology*, *9*(6), 1087–1101. doi:10.1037/0022-3514.92.6.1087 PMID:17547490

Fink, J. E. (2014). Flourishing: Exploring predictors of mental health within the college environment. *Journal of American College Health*, *62*(6), 380–388. doi:10.1080/07448481.2014.917647 PMID:24779485

National Alliance on Mental Illness. (2016). *Starting the conversation: College and your mental health.* Retrieved April 11, 2017, from https://www.nami.org/collegeguide/download

Related Readings

To continue IGI Global's long-standing tradition of advancing innovation through emerging research, please find below a compiled list of recommended IGI Global book chapters and journal articles in the areas of mental health, academic stress, and intellectual disabilities. These related readings will provide additional information and guidance to further enrich your knowledge and assist you with your own research.

Akbar, S., & Khurana, H. (2017). Chronic Mental Illness in Old Age Homes: An International Perspective. In B. Prasad (Ed.), *Chronic Mental Illness and the Changing Scope of Intervention Strategies, Diagnosis, and Treatment* (pp. 21–39). Hershey, PA: IGI Global. doi:10.4018/978-1-5225-0519-8.ch002

Al Ja'am, J. M., Abou El-Seoud, M. S., Dandashi, A., & Karkar, A. (2016). A Cognitive and Augmentative Communication System for Special Needs Education. In M. Gordon (Ed.), *Challenges Surrounding the Education of Children with Chronic Diseases* (pp. 323–342). Hershey, PA: IGI Global. doi:10.4018/978-1-4666-9452-1.ch015

Amos, Y. T. (2016). Guest Students: Faculty Expectations of Japanese International Students. In K. Bista & C. Foster (Eds.), *Exploring the Social and Academic Experiences of International Students in Higher Education Institutions* (pp. 260–291). Hershey, PA: IGI Global. doi:10.4018/978-1-4666-9749-2.ch014

Andersson, F., & Sundh, S. (2015). Young Learners: Communication and Digital Tools. In T. Hansson (Ed.), *Contemporary Approaches to Activity Theory: Interdisciplinary Perspectives on Human Behavior* (pp. 19–37). Hershey, PA: IGI Global. doi:10.4018/978-1-4666-6603-0.ch002

Andreasen, K. E., & Rasmussen, P. (2015). Learning in Video-Mediated Classes. In T. Hansson (Ed.), *Contemporary Approaches to Activity Theory: Interdisciplinary Perspectives on Human Behavior* (pp. 38–53). Hershey, PA: IGI Global. doi:10.4018/978-1-4666-6603-0.ch003

Arden, M., Manathunga, C., & Bottrell, D. (2017). Internationalisation and Identity: Identity Construction Through Australian University Student Mobility Program. In A. Shahriar & G. Syed (Eds.), *Student Culture and Identity in Higher Education* (pp. 1–17). Hershey, PA: IGI Global. doi:10.4018/978-1-5225-2551-6.ch001

Athota, V. S. (2017). Foundations and Future of Well-Being: How Personality Influences Happiness and Well-Being. In S. Háša & R. Brunet-Thornton (Eds.), *Impact of Organizational Trauma on Workplace Behavior and Performance* (pp. 279–294). Hershey, PA: IGI Global. doi:10.4018/978-1-5225-2021-4.ch012

B. N. R., Prasad, B. V., & Tavaragi, M. S. (2017). Legal Aspects of Chronic Mental Illness. In B. Prasad (Ed.), Chronic Mental Illness and the Changing Scope of Intervention Strategies, Diagnosis, and Treatment (pp. 225-235). Hershey, PA: IGI Global. doi:10.4018/978-1-5225-0519-8.ch012

Bang, L. (2015). Mapping [Capital v.2.0]: An Encounter of Thoughts. In T. Hansson (Ed.), Contemporary Approaches to Activity Theory: Interdisciplinary Perspectives on Human Behavior (pp. 337-352). Hershey, PA: IGI Global. doi:10.4018/978-1-4666-6603-0.ch020

Banks, S. (2017). Mirrors of Opportunity: Joint Project of Japanese and International Students. In A. Shahriar & G. Syed (Eds.), *Student Culture and Identity in Higher Education* (pp. 18–37). Hershey, PA: IGI Global. doi:10.4018/978-1-5225-2551-6.ch002

Bedi, D. (2017). Efficacy of Art Therapy in Treating Patients with Paranoid Schizophrenia. In B. Prasad (Ed.), *Chronic Mental Illness and the Changing Scope of Intervention Strategies, Diagnosis, and Treatment* (pp. 308–320). Hershey, PA: IGI Global. doi:10.4018/978-1-5225-0519-8.ch017

Behrani, P., & Deka, D. B. (2016). Concerns for Individuals with Intellectual Disability in India. In R. Gopalan (Ed.), *Handbook of Research on Diagnosing, Treating, and Managing Intellectual Disabilities* (pp. 204–219). Hershey, PA: IGI Global. doi:10.4018/978-1-5225-0089-6.ch011

Bhargava, S., & Umrigar, D. M. (2016). Intellectual Disability in the Family Context: Parents with Intellectual Disability. In R. Gopalan (Ed.), *Handbook of Research on Diagnosing, Treating, and Managing Intellectual Disabilities* (pp. 370–385). Hershey, PA: IGI Global. doi:10.4018/978-1-5225-0089-6.ch019

Billington, R. (2017). A Critique on the Factors that Influence Mental Health Workforce Training in Developing Countries. In M. Smith & A. Jury (Eds.), *Workforce Development Theory and Practice in the Mental Health Sector* (pp. 130–143). Hershey, PA: IGI Global. doi:10.4018/978-1-5225-1874-7.ch006

Bingham, H. M. (2017). Undergraduate Nursing Curriculum Content Focuses on Emerging Issues that Influence Health. In M. Smith & A. Jury (Eds.), *Workforce Development Theory and Practice in the Mental Health Sector* (pp. 182–199). Hershey, PA: IGI Global. doi:10.4018/978-1-5225-1874-7.ch009

Bordoloi, S. D. (2016). Addressing the Needs of F-2 Wives in the United States: A Comparison of Two Educational Institutions. In K. Bista & C. Foster (Eds.), *Exploring the Social and Academic Experiences of International Students in Higher Education Institutions* (pp. 115–131). Hershey, PA: IGI Global. doi:10.4018/978-1-4666-9749-2.ch007

Bunda, T., Qi, J., Manathunga, C., & Singh, M. J. (2017). Enhancing the Australian Doctoral Experience: Locating Culture and Identity at the Centre. In A. Shahriar & G. Syed (Eds.), *Student Culture and Identity in Higher Education* (pp. 143–159). Hershey, PA: IGI Global. doi:10.4018/978-1-5225-2551-6.ch009

Byrd-Poller, L., Farmer, J. L., & Ford, V. (2017). The Role of Leaders in Facilitating Healing After Organizational Trauma. In S. Háša & R. Brunet-Thornton (Eds.), *Impact of Organizational Trauma on Workplace Behavior and Performance* (pp. 318–340). Hershey, PA: IGI Global. doi:10.4018/978-1-5225-2021-4.ch014

Cejka, P., & Mohelska, H. (2017). National Culture Influence on Organisational Trauma: A Conceptual Framework Review. In S. Háša & R. Brunet-Thornton (Eds.), *Impact of Organizational Trauma on Workplace Behavior and Performance* (pp. 162–186). Hershey, PA: IGI Global. doi:10.4018/978-1-5225-2021-4.ch007

Chen, B., & Luppicini, R. (2017). The New Era of Bullying: A Phenomenological Study of University Students Past Experience with Cyberbullying. *International Journal of Cyber Behavior, Psychology and Learning*, 7(2), 72–90. doi:10.4018/IJCBPL.2017040106

Chowhan, S., & Patowary, P. (2016). Issues and Recent Trends in the Assessment and Management of ID in Childhood. In R. Gopalan (Ed.), *Handbook of Research on Diagnosing, Treating, and Managing Intellectual Disabilities* (pp. 186–203). Hershey, PA: IGI Global. doi:10.4018/978-1-5225-0089-6.ch010

Cleve, R. A., Işık, İ., & Pecanha, V. D. (2017). Sexual Identities in the Workplace: Avoiding Organizational Trauma When Disclosure Occurs – Current Perspectives. In S. Háša & R. Brunet-Thornton (Eds.), *Impact of Organizational Trauma on Workplace Behavior and Performance* (pp. 188–220). Hershey, PA: IGI Global. doi:10.4018/978-1-5225-2021-4.ch008

Cook, B. L. (2016). Effectively Teaching Stressed Students. In K. Pandey & P. Upadhyay (Eds.), *Promoting Global Peace and Civic Engagement through Education* (pp. 228–241). Hershey, PA: IGI Global. doi:10.4018/978-1-5225-0078-0.ch013

Coombs, T., Burgess, P., Dickson, R., & McKay, R. (2017). Routine Outcome Measurement and the Development of the Australian Mental Health Workforce: The First 25 Years of Implementation Are the Hardest. In M. Smith & A. Jury (Eds.), *Workforce Development Theory and Practice in the Mental Health Sector* (pp. 302–316). Hershey, PA: IGI Global. doi:10.4018/978-1-5225-1874-7.ch015

Dang, C. T., & Kline, S. L. (2015). "I Can't Afford for You to Flunk": Positive Asian Stereotypes and Supportive Communication for Asian College Students. In N. Hartlep (Ed.), *Modern Societal Impacts of the Model Minority Stereotype* (pp. 1–34). Hershey, PA: IGI Global. doi:10.4018/978-1-4666-7467-7.ch001

de Soir, E., & Kleber, R. (2017). Understanding the Core of Psychological Trauma: Trauma in Contemporary French Theory. In S. Háša & R. Brunet-Thornton (Eds.), *Impact of Organizational Trauma on Workplace Behavior and Performance* (pp. 57–75). Hershey, PA: IGI Global. doi:10.4018/978-1-5225-2021-4.ch003

Dehuri, B. K., & Mukund, B. (2016). Recent Trends and Issues in Vocational Rehabilitation of People with ID. In R. Gopalan (Ed.), *Handbook of Research on Diagnosing, Treating, and Managing Intellectual Disabilities* (pp. 283–309). Hershey, PA: IGI Global. doi:10.4018/978-1-5225-0089-6.ch015

Dixon, K. V., Gonzalez-Carriedo, R., & Dixon-Krauss, L. (2017). The Implementation and Analysis of an International Student Teaching Program. In L. Leavitt, S. Wisdom, & K. Leavitt (Eds.), *Cultural Awareness and Competency Development in Higher Education* (pp. 168–188). Hershey, PA: IGI Global. doi:10.4018/978-1-5225-2145-7.ch010

Dorado, D. A., & Fass-Holmes, B. (2016). Academic Achievement and Demographics of International Undergraduates. In K. Bista & C. Foster (Eds.), *Exploring the Social and Academic Experiences of International Students in Higher Education Institutions* (pp. 233–259). Hershey, PA: IGI Global. doi:10.4018/978-1-4666-9749-2.ch013

Eapen, V., & Walter, A. (2016). Mind the Gap: Developmental Vulnerability and Mental Health. In R. Gopalan (Ed.), *Handbook of Research on Diagnosing, Treating, and Managing Intellectual Disabilities* (pp. 11–32). Hershey, PA: IGI Global. doi:10.4018/978-1-5225-0089-6.ch002

Enerstvedt, R. T. (2015). Reflections on the Theory of Activity. In T. Hansson (Ed.), *Contemporary Approaches to Activity Theory: Interdisciplinary Perspectives on Human Behavior* (pp. 353–363). Hershey, PA: IGI Global. doi:10.4018/978-1-4666-6603-0.ch021

Eriksson, I. (2015). Constitution of Objects in DWR Activity. In T. Hansson (Ed.), *Contemporary Approaches to Activity Theory: Interdisciplinary Perspectives on Human Behavior* (pp. 304–321). Hershey, PA: IGI Global. doi:10.4018/978-1-4666-6603-0.ch018

Farrell, H. J. (2016). Imagining Social Equity. In M. Gordon (Ed.), *Challenges Surrounding the Education of Children with Chronic Diseases* (pp. 247–261). Hershey, PA: IGI Global. doi:10.4018/978-1-4666-9452-1.ch012

Fellus, O. O., & Fellus, D. P. (2016). Living with ADHD: Timing Perceptions and Their Applicability to the Experience of ADHD. In M. Gordon (Ed.), *Challenges Surrounding the Education of Children with Chronic Diseases* (pp. 117–136). Hershey, PA: IGI Global. doi:10.4018/978-1-4666-9452-1.ch006

Fellus, Y. M., & Fellus, I. A. (2016). The Experience of Cancer and Asthma in the Pediatric Patient: A Family Physician's Perspective. In M. Gordon (Ed.), *Challenges Surrounding the Education of Children with Chronic Diseases* (pp. 12–25). Hershey, PA: IGI Global. doi:10.4018/978-1-4666-9452-1.ch002

Ferholt, B., Nilsson, M., Jansson, A., & Alnervik, K. (2015). Creativity in Education: Play and Exploratory Learning. In T. Hansson (Ed.), *Contemporary Approaches to Activity Theory: Interdisciplinary Perspectives on Human Behavior* (pp. 264–284). Hershey, PA: IGI Global. doi:10.4018/978-1-4666-6603-0.ch016

Firdaus, J., & Jadeja, M. (2016). Quality of Life of People with Intellectual Disability. In R. Gopalan (Ed.), *Handbook of Research on Diagnosing, Treating, and Managing Intellectual Disabilities* (pp. 139–155). Hershey, PA: IGI Global. doi:10.4018/978-1-5225-0089-6.ch008

G., L. (2017). Psychosocial Intervention Studies for Street Children with Substance Abuse. In B. Prasad (Ed.), *Chronic Mental Illness and the Changing Scope of Intervention Strategies, Diagnosis, and Treatment* (pp. 237-257). Hershey, PA: IGI Global. doi:10.4018/978-1-5225-0519-8.ch013

Gallego, J. (2017). Organizational Trauma and Change Management. In S. Háša & R. Brunet-Thornton (Eds.), *Impact of Organizational Trauma on Workplace Behavior and Performance* (pp. 140–161). Hershey, PA: IGI Global. doi:10.4018/978-1-5225-2021-4.ch006

García-Sánchez, S., & Hernández-Guerra, C. (2017). Academic ESP Oral Production: Moving Forward Towards Local and Global Awareness. In L. Leavitt, S. Wisdom, & K. Leavitt (Eds.), *Cultural Awareness and Competency Development in Higher Education* (pp. 255–271). Hershey, PA: IGI Global. doi:10.4018/978-1-5225-2145-7.ch015

Garg, B., Khanna, P., & Khanna, A. (2017). Chronic Mental Illness and the Changing Scope of Intervention Strategies, Diagnosis, and Treatment in Child and Adolescent Population. In B. Prasad (Ed.), *Chronic Mental Illness and the Changing Scope of Intervention Strategies, Diagnosis, and Treatment* (pp. 258–269). Hershey, PA: IGI Global. doi:10.4018/978-1-5225-0519-8.ch014

Ghosh, N., Sinha, V. K., & Poddar, S. (2016). Vocational Rehabilitation: Recent Trends and Issues in Vocational Rehabilitation of People with ID. In R. Gopalan (Ed.), *Handbook of Research on Diagnosing, Treating, and Managing Intellectual Disabilities* (pp. 310–330). Hershey, PA: IGI Global. doi:10.4018/978-1-5225-0089-6.ch016

Giannouli, V. (2016). Crime and Legal Issues among Intellectually Disabled Individuals. In R. Gopalan (Ed.), *Handbook of Research on Diagnosing, Treating, and Managing Intellectual Disabilities* (pp. 346–369). Hershey, PA: IGI Global. doi:10.4018/978-1-5225-0089-6.ch018

Gibbon, M., Duffy, C. M., Taylor, G., & Laniel, S. (2016). Juvenile Idiopathic Arthritis (JIA) and Education in Primary School Children. In M. Gordon (Ed.), *Challenges Surrounding the Education of Children with Chronic Diseases* (pp. 59–84). Hershey, PA: IGI Global. doi:10.4018/978-1-4666-9452-1.ch004

Gibbon, T. C., Cline, J., Schwilk, C. L., Hosfelt, P. D., & Bateman, D. F. (2016). The Educational Rights of Students with Chronic Disease. In M. Gordon (Ed.), *Challenges Surrounding the Education of Children with Chronic Diseases* (pp. 199–226). Hershey, PA: IGI Global. doi:10.4018/978-1-4666-9452-1.ch010

Gibbon, T. C., Schwilk, C. L., Cline, J., Matthews, K., Sweigart, K., Ferguson, E., & Bateman, D. F. (2016). Case Studies of Chronically Ill Children: Implications for Education Professionals. In M. Gordon (Ed.), *Challenges Surrounding the Education of Children with Chronic Diseases* (pp. 263–296). Hershey, PA: IGI Global. doi:10.4018/978-1-4666-9452-1.ch013

Gopal, A. (2016). Academic Experiences of International Graduate Students: The Canadian Perspective in the Context of Internationalization. In K. Bista & C. Foster (Eds.), *Exploring the Social and Academic Experiences of International Students in Higher Education Institutions* (pp. 21–37). Hershey, PA: IGI Global. doi:10.4018/978-1-4666-9749-2.ch002

Gopalan, R. T. (2016). Intellectual Disability: From History to Recent Trends. In R. Gopalan (Ed.), *Handbook of Research on Diagnosing, Treating, and Managing Intellectual Disabilities* (pp. 1–10). Hershey, PA: IGI Global. doi:10.4018/978-1-5225-0089-6.ch001

Gopalan, R. T., & Agustus, P. (2016). Sexuality, Parenting Skills, and Related Issues in Persons with Intellectual Disability. In R. Gopalan (Ed.), *Handbook of Research on Diagnosing, Treating, and Managing Intellectual Disabilities* (pp. 386–395). Hershey, PA: IGI Global. doi:10.4018/978-1-5225-0089-6.ch020

Gordon, M. (2016). Parents as Advocates for Children with IBD at School. In M. Gordon (Ed.), *Challenges Surrounding the Education of Children with Chronic Diseases* (pp. 138–150). Hershey, PA: IGI Global. doi:10.4018/978-1-4666-9452-1.ch007

Gordon, M. (2016). The School Experiences of Children with Inflammatory Bowel Disease. In M. Gordon (Ed.), *Challenges Surrounding the Education of Children with Chronic Diseases* (pp. 1–11). Hershey, PA: IGI Global. doi:10.4018/978-1-4666-9452-1.ch001

Graham, D., Killoran, I., & Parekh, G. (2016). Supporting Students' Mental Health and Emotional Well-Being in Inclusive Classrooms. In M. Gordon (Ed.), *Challenges Surrounding the Education of Children with Chronic Diseases* (pp. 86–116). Hershey, PA: IGI Global. doi:10.4018/978-1-4666-9452-1.ch005

Green, W. M., & De Cruz, V. (2017). Enhancing Intercultural Competency Though Co-Curricular Activities in Higher Education: Three Examples From an American University. In A. Shahriar & G. Syed (Eds.), *Student Culture and Identity in Higher Education* (pp. 59–74). Hershey, PA: IGI Global. doi:10.4018/978-1-5225-2551-6.ch004

Gupta, S. K. (2016). Use of Assistive Technology to Empower Persons with Intellectual Disabilities. In R. Gopalan (Ed.), *Handbook of Research on Diagnosing, Treating, and Managing Intellectual Disabilities* (pp. 331–345). Hershey, PA: IGI Global. doi:10.4018/978-1-5225-0089-6.ch017

Halder, S., & Mahato, A. (2017). Cognitive Remediation Therapy in Chronic Schizophrenia. In B. Prasad (Ed.), *Chronic Mental Illness and the Changing Scope of Intervention Strategies, Diagnosis, and Treatment* (pp. 292–307). Hershey, PA: IGI Global. doi:10.4018/978-1-5225-0519-8.ch016

Hansson, T. (2015). Modeling and Analyzing Contextual Influences. In T. Hansson (Ed.), *Contemporary Approaches to Activity Theory: Interdisciplinary Perspectives on Human Behavior* (pp. 249–263). Hershey, PA: IGI Global. doi:10.4018/978-1-4666-6603-0.ch015

Hart, A., Lantz, C., & Montague, J. (2017). Identity, Power, and Discomfort: Developing Intercultural Competence Through Transformative Learning. In A. Shahriar & G. Syed (Eds.), *Student Culture and Identity in Higher Education* (pp. 38–58). Hershey, PA: IGI Global. doi:10.4018/978-1-5225-2551-6.ch003

Hashim, A. H., Kaur, M., Bahar, N., & Ismail, W. S. (2016). Mental Health Issues among Family Members of Children with Mental Disability. In R. Gopalan (Ed.), *Handbook of Research on Diagnosing, Treating, and Managing Intellectual Disabilities* (pp. 54–81). Hershey, PA: IGI Global. doi:10.4018/978-1-5225-0089-6.ch004

Hazarika, M., & Choudhury, S. (2016). Attitude towards People with Intellectual Disabilities (PWID). In R. Gopalan (Ed.), *Handbook of Research on Diagnosing, Treating, and Managing Intellectual Disabilities* (pp. 237–261). Hershey, PA: IGI Global. doi:10.4018/978-1-5225-0089-6.ch013

Hennessy, J. L., Smythe, L., Abbott, M., & Hughes, F. A. (2017). Mental Health Support Workers: An Evolving Workforce. In M. Smith & A. Jury (Eds.), *Workforce Development Theory and Practice in the Mental Health Sector* (pp. 200–221). Hershey, PA: IGI Global. doi:10.4018/978-1-5225-1874-7.ch010

Hill, C. W., & Withy, K. (2017). Rural Mental Health Workforce Development in Hawai'i and the US-Affiliated Pacific Islands. In M. Smith & A. Jury (Eds.), *Workforce Development Theory and Practice in the Mental Health Sector* (pp. 60–89). Hershey, PA: IGI Global. doi:10.4018/978-1-5225-1874-7.ch003

Hoffman, J. C., & Osipoff, J. N. (2016). Type 1 Diabetes Mellitus in the Inclusive School Setting: Daily and Long Term Effects on Education. In M. Gordon (Ed.), *Challenges Surrounding the Education of Children with Chronic Diseases* (pp. 26–58). Hershey, PA: IGI Global. doi:10.4018/978-1-4666-9452-1.ch003

Hoge, M. A., Stuart, G. W., Morris, J. A., Huey, L. Y., Flaherty, M. T., & Paris, M. Jr. (2017). Behavioral Health Workforce Development in the United States. In M. Smith & A. Jury (Eds.), *Workforce Development Theory and Practice in the Mental Health Sector* (pp. 37–59). Hershey, PA: IGI Global. doi:10.4018/978-1-5225-1874-7.ch002

Huda, M., Sabani, N., Shahrill, M., Jasmi, K. A., Basiron, B., & Mustari, M. I. (2017). Empowering Learning Culture as Student Identity Construction in Higher Education. In A. Shahriar & G. Syed (Eds.), *Student Culture and Identity in Higher Education* (pp. 160–179). Hershey, PA: IGI Global. doi:10.4018/978-1-5225-2551-6.ch010

Isik, I. (2017). Organizations and Exposure to Trauma at a Collective Level: The Taxonomy of Potentially Traumatic Events. In S. Háša & R. Brunet-Thornton (Eds.), *Impact of Organizational Trauma on Workplace Behavior and Performance* (pp. 18–56). Hershey, PA: IGI Global. doi:10.4018/978-1-5225-2021-4.ch002

Islam, S. M., Tabassum, R., Colet, P. C., Cruz, J. P., Dey, S., Rawal, L. B., & Islam, A. (2017). Human Resources for Mental Health in Low and Middle Income Countries: Evidence from Bangladesh. In M. Smith & A. Jury (Eds.), *Workforce Development Theory and Practice in the Mental Health Sector* (pp. 144–164). Hershey, PA: IGI Global. doi:10.4018/978-1-5225-1874-7.ch007

Janus, M., & Siddiqua, A. (2016). Challenges for Children with Special Health Needs at the Time of Transition to School. In M. Gordon (Ed.), *Challenges Surrounding the Education of Children with Chronic Diseases* (pp. 165–197). Hershey, PA: IGI Global. doi:10.4018/978-1-4666-9452-1.ch009

Jerabek, I., & Muoio, D. (2017). The Stress Profile: The Influence of Personal Characteristics on Response to Occupational Trauma. In S. Háša & R. Brunet-Thornton (Eds.), *Impact of Organizational Trauma on Workplace Behavior and Performance* (pp. 77–119). Hershey, PA: IGI Global. doi:10.4018/978-1-5225-2021-4.ch004

Jha, S., Khanna, A., & Khanna, P. (2017). Advanced Intervention Strategies for Suicide in Patients with Chronic Mental Illness. In B. Prasad (Ed.), *Chronic Mental Illness and the Changing Scope of Intervention Strategies, Diagnosis, and Treatment* (pp. 271–291). Hershey, PA: IGI Global. doi:10.4018/978-1-5225-0519-8.ch015

Jóhannsdóttir, T. (2015). Responsive Practices in Online Teacher Education. In T. Hansson (Ed.), *Contemporary Approaches to Activity Theory: Interdisciplinary Perspectives on Human Behavior* (pp. 1–18). Hershey, PA: IGI Global. doi:10.4018/978-1-4666-6603-0.ch001

Johansson, K. (2015). Collaborative Music Making and Artistic Agency. In T. Hansson (Ed.), *Contemporary Approaches to Activity Theory: Interdisciplinary Perspectives on Human Behavior* (pp. 73–91). Hershey, PA: IGI Global. doi:10.4018/978-1-4666-6603-0.ch005

Jonasson, C. (2015). Vocational Learning Mediated by Constructive Competition. In T. Hansson (Ed.), *Contemporary Approaches to Activity Theory: Interdisciplinary Perspectives on Human Behavior* (pp. 92–107). Hershey, PA: IGI Global. doi:10.4018/978-1-4666-6603-0.ch006

Kakkori, L., & Huttunen, R. (2015). Vygotsky, Heidegger, and Gadamer on Moral Development. In T. Hansson (Ed.), *Contemporary Approaches to Activity Theory: Interdisciplinary Perspectives on Human Behavior* (pp. 323–336). Hershey, PA: IGI Global. doi:10.4018/978-1-4666-6603-0.ch019

Kaushik, P., & Singh, T. B. (2017). Predictors of Expressed Emotion, Caregiver's Burden, and Quality of Life in Chronic Mental Illness. In B. Prasad (Ed.), *Chronic Mental Illness and the Changing Scope of Intervention Strategies, Diagnosis, and Treatment* (pp. 143–163). Hershey, PA: IGI Global. doi:10.4018/978-1-5225-0519-8.ch008

Kennedy, B. F., & McLaughlin, P. M. (2017). Growing Global STEM Learning in Higher Education. In L. Leavitt, S. Wisdom, & K. Leavitt (Eds.), *Cultural Awareness and Competency Development in Higher Education* (pp. 132–147). Hershey, PA: IGI Global. doi:10.4018/978-1-5225-2145-7.ch008

Kılıç, B. (2017). An Organizational Trauma Intervention: A Case From Turkey. In S. Háša & R. Brunet-Thornton (Eds.), *Impact of Organizational Trauma on Workplace Behavior and Performance* (pp. 264–277). Hershey, PA: IGI Global. doi:10.4018/978-1-5225-2021-4.ch011

Kim, Y. K., Carter, J. L., & Armstrong, C. L. (2017). Civic Responsibility Development Among College Students: How Is It Different by Student Race? In L. Leavitt, S. Wisdom, & K. Leavitt (Eds.), *Cultural Awareness and Competency Development in Higher Education* (pp. 92–110). Hershey, PA: IGI Global. doi:10.4018/978-1-5225-2145-7.ch006

Koning, A., & Poole, S. J. (2017). Supporting People Who Experience Co-Existing Mental Health and Addiction Problems: A National Approach to Improving Responsiveness in Aotearoa New Zealand. In M. Smith & A. Jury (Eds.), *Workforce Development Theory and Practice in the Mental Health Sector* (pp. 251–270). Hershey, PA: IGI Global. doi:10.4018/978-1-5225-1874-7.ch012

Kučera, D. (2017). The Potential of Spirituality for the Treatment of Organizational Trauma. In S. Háša & R. Brunet-Thornton (Eds.), *Impact of Organizational Trauma on Workplace Behavior and Performance* (pp. 295–317). Hershey, PA: IGI Global. doi:10.4018/978-1-5225-2021-4.ch013

Kukreti, P., Khanna, P., & Khanna, A. (2017). Chronic Mental Illnesses and Homelessness. In B. Prasad (Ed.), *Chronic Mental Illness and the Changing Scope of Intervention Strategies, Diagnosis, and Treatment* (pp. 1–20). Hershey, PA: IGI Global. doi:10.4018/978-1-5225-0519-8.ch001

Kyhlbäck, H. (2015). Game Construction Activity in Higher Education. In T. Hansson (Ed.), *Contemporary Approaches to Activity Theory: Interdisciplinary Perspectives on Human Behavior* (pp. 54–71). Hershey, PA: IGI Global. doi:10.4018/978-1-4666-6603-0.ch004

Laffier, J., Petrarca, D., & Hughes, J. M. (2017). The Need for Promoting and Developing Cultural Competency in Future Teachers. In L. Leavitt, S. Wisdom, & K. Leavitt (Eds.), *Cultural Awareness and Competency Development in Higher Education* (pp. 148–167). Hershey, PA: IGI Global. doi:10.4018/978-1-5225-2145-7.ch009

Lawson, R., & Dunnachie, B. (2017). Workforce Development in the Child and Adolescent Mental Health Sector: The Challenge of Rolling out a Specialist Eating Disorders Treatment in New Zealand. In M. Smith & A. Jury (Eds.), *Workforce Development Theory and Practice in the Mental Health Sector* (pp. 271–283). Hershey, PA: IGI Global. doi:10.4018/978-1-5225-1874-7.ch013

Lewis, A. (2016). Making Meaning of Race and Racialization in the Lives of Five International Graduate Students. In K. Bista & C. Foster (Eds.), *Exploring the Social and Academic Experiences of International Students in Higher Education Institutions* (pp. 59–78). Hershey, PA: IGI Global. doi:10.4018/978-1-4666-9749-2.ch004

Li, M. (2016). Learning the Rules of the Game: Issues Affecting Academic Acculturation of Asian International Students in New Zealand Universities. In K. Bista & C. Foster (Eds.), *Exploring the Social and Academic Experiences of International Students in Higher Education Institutions* (pp. 38–58). Hershey, PA: IGI Global. doi:10.4018/978-1-4666-9749-2.ch003

Lin, X., & Baker, B. A. (2017). Challenges and Changing Attitudes for Chinese Women Seeking PhDs. In A. Shahriar & G. Syed (Eds.), *Student Culture and Identity in Higher Education* (pp. 76–92). Hershey, PA: IGI Global. doi:10.4018/978-1-5225-2551-6.ch005

Linge, A. (2015). Creative Musical Practice in an Educational Context. In T. Hansson (Ed.), *Contemporary Approaches to Activity Theory: Interdisciplinary Perspectives on Human Behavior* (pp. 143–160). Hershey, PA: IGI Global. doi:10.4018/978-1-4666-6603-0.ch009

M., K., & Boominathan, P. (2016). Assessment and Management of Communication Skills in Individuals with Intellectual Disability: Perspectives in the 21st Century. In R. Gopalan (Ed.), *Handbook of Research on Diagnosing, Treating, and Managing Intellectual Disabilities* (pp. 156-185). Hershey, PA: IGI Global. doi:10.4018/978-1-5225-0089-6.ch009

Mahato, A., & Halder, S. (2017). Disability in Schizophrenia: The Psychosocial and Neurocognitive Perspective. In B. Prasad (Ed.), *Chronic Mental Illness and the Changing Scope of Intervention Strategies, Diagnosis, and Treatment* (pp. 188–202). Hershey, PA: IGI Global. doi:10.4018/978-1-5225-0519-8.ch010

Maich, K., Belcher, C., Sider, S., & Johnson, N. (2016). Using Children's Literature to Support Social-Emotional Growth in the Classroom: A Bibliotherapeutic Approach to Education about Chronic Disease. In M. Gordon (Ed.), *Challenges Surrounding the Education of Children with Chronic Diseases* (pp. 297–322). Hershey, PA: IGI Global. doi:10.4018/978-1-4666-9452-1.ch014

Manguvo, A. (2016). Negotiating the Boundaries of American Blackness: The Experiences of African Students in the United States. In K. Bista & C. Foster (Eds.), *Exploring the Social and Academic Experiences of International Students in Higher Education Institutions* (pp. 79–95). Hershey, PA: IGI Global. doi:10.4018/978-1-4666-9749-2.ch005

Martin, K. J. (2017). International Students in Higher Education: More Than a Fish Out of Water. In L. Leavitt, S. Wisdom, & K. Leavitt (Eds.), *Cultural Awareness and Competency Development in Higher Education* (pp. 21–39). Hershey, PA: IGI Global. doi:10.4018/978-1-5225-2145-7.ch002

McKay, R., Coombs, T., & Anderson, J. M. (2017). Mental Health and Addiction Workforce Development in Australia: Never the Twain to Meet? In M. Smith & A. Jury (Eds.), *Workforce Development Theory and Practice in the Mental Health Sector* (pp. 90–105). Hershey, PA: IGI Global. doi:10.4018/978-1-5225-1874-7.ch004

McMillan, S. J., & Ripley, C. D. (2017). Persistence Profiles and Institutional Initiatives: Helping Students Become Ready for the World. In L. Leavitt, S. Wisdom, & K. Leavitt (Eds.), *Cultural Awareness and Competency Development in Higher Education* (pp. 288–303). Hershey, PA: IGI Global. doi:10.4018/978-1-5225-2145-7.ch017

Mueller, C., King, M. D., & Klar, D. (2017). Reframing White Privilege. In L. Leavitt, S. Wisdom, & K. Leavitt (Eds.), *Cultural Awareness and Competency Development in Higher Education* (pp. 61–74). Hershey, PA: IGI Global. doi:10.4018/978-1-5225-2145-7.ch004

Mugambwa, J., Mwebaza, S., & Namubiru, B. (2017). Gender Equality Policy, Elites and Women Empowerment in Higher Education Institutions. In A. Shahriar & G. Syed (Eds.), *Student Culture and Identity in Higher Education* (pp. 93–110). Hershey, PA: IGI Global. doi:10.4018/978-1-5225-2551-6.ch006

Mwangi, C. A., Peralta, A. M., Fries-Britt, S., & Daoud, N. (2016). Academic Motivation and Experiences of International Students of Color in STEM. In K. Bista & C. Foster (Eds.), *Exploring the Social and Academic Experiences of International Students in Higher Education Institutions* (pp. 197–211). Hershey, PA: IGI Global. doi:10.4018/978-1-4666-9749-2.ch011

Myers, Z. R., Swearer, S. M., Martin, M. J., & Palacios, R. (2017). Cyberbullying and Traditional Bullying: The Experiences of Poly-Victimization Among Diverse Youth. *International Journal of Technoethics*, *8*(2), 42–60. doi:10.4018/IJT.2017070104

Nascimento, C. P. (2015). Subject Matter Analysis in Physical Education. In T. Hansson (Ed.), *Contemporary Approaches to Activity Theory: Interdisciplinary Perspectives on Human Behavior* (pp. 229–248). Hershey, PA: IGI Global. doi:10.4018/978-1-4666-6603-0.ch014

Pandey, J. M., & Mishra, P. (2016). Intellectual Disability: An Awareness towards Intervention. In R. Gopalan (Ed.), *Handbook of Research on Diagnosing, Treating, and Managing Intellectual Disabilities* (pp. 220–236). Hershey, PA: IGI Global. doi:10.4018/978-1-5225-0089-6.ch012

Pandey, J. M., Mishra, P., Garg, S., & Mshra, B. P. (2017). Chronic Mental Illness and Dumping Patients: A Concern towards Management. In B. Prasad (Ed.), *Chronic Mental Illness and the Changing Scope of Intervention Strategies, Diagnosis, and Treatment* (pp. 40–57). Hershey, PA: IGI Global. doi:10.4018/978-1-5225-0519-8.ch003

Pena, P. A., Van den Broucke, S., Sylin, M., Leysen, J., & de Soir, E. (2017). Definitions, Typologies, and Processes Involved in Organizational Trauma: A Literature Review. In S. Háša & R. Brunet-Thornton (Eds.), *Impact of Organizational Trauma on Workplace Behavior and Performance* (pp. 1–17). Hershey, PA: IGI Global. doi:10.4018/978-1-5225-2021-4.ch001

Popov, O. (2015). Outdoor Science in Teacher Education. In T. Hansson (Ed.), *Contemporary Approaches to Activity Theory: Interdisciplinary Perspectives on Human Behavior* (pp. 128–142). Hershey, PA: IGI Global. doi:10.4018/978-1-4666-6603-0.ch008

Prusty, B. (2016). The Stress and Adjustment in the Family of Intellectually Disabled Children. In R. Gopalan (Ed.), *Handbook of Research on Diagnosing, Treating, and Managing Intellectual Disabilities* (pp. 82–108). Hershey, PA: IGI Global. doi:10.4018/978-1-5225-0089-6.ch005

Pulotu-Endemann, F. K., & Faleafa, M. (2017). Developing a Culturally Competent Workforce that Meets the Needs of Pacific People Living in New Zealand. In M. Smith & A. Jury (Eds.), *Workforce Development Theory and Practice in the Mental Health Sector* (pp. 165–180). Hershey, PA: IGI Global. doi:10.4018/978-1-5225-1874-7.ch008

R., A., Prasad, B. V., & Kosgi, S. (2017). Psychosocial Intervention Strategies for Patients with Schizophrenia: In Chronic Mental Illness. In B. Prasad (Ed.), *Chronic Mental Illness and the Changing Scope of Intervention Strategies, Diagnosis, and Treatment* (pp. 58-75). Hershey, PA: IGI Global. doi:10.4018/978-1-5225-0519-8.ch004

Raghunandan-Jack, N. (2017). Teacher Preparatory Programs and Culturally Responsive Teaching. In L. Leavitt, S. Wisdom, & K. Leavitt (Eds.), *Cultural Awareness and Competency Development in Higher Education* (pp. 207–222). Hershey, PA: IGI Global. doi:10.4018/978-1-5225-2145-7.ch012

Rell, A. B., Puig, R. A., Roll, F., Valles, V., Espinoza, M., & Duque, A. L. (2017). Addressing Cultural Diversity and Global Competence: The Dual Language Framework. In L. Leavitt, S. Wisdom, & K. Leavitt (Eds.), *Cultural Awareness and Competency Development in Higher Education* (pp. 111–131). Hershey, PA: IGI Global. doi:10.4018/978-1-5225-2145-7.ch007

Ristimäki, P. (2015). Explorative Actions in Search for a New Logic of Business Activity. In T. Hansson (Ed.), *Contemporary Approaches to Activity Theory: Interdisciplinary Perspectives on Human Behavior* (pp. 181–197). Hershey, PA: IGI Global. doi:10.4018/978-1-4666-6603-0.ch011

Ritter, Z. S. (2016). Globalization of Racism: Chinese, Japanese, and Korean International Students' Racial Stereotypes and Experiences with Cross-Racial Interactions. In K. Bista & C. Foster (Eds.), *Exploring the Social and Academic Experiences of International Students in Higher Education Institutions* (pp. 132–155). Hershey, PA: IGI Global. doi:10.4018/978-1-4666-9749-2.ch008

Roche, A. M., & Nicholas, R. S. (2017). Mental Health and Addictions Workforce Development: Past, Present, and Future. In M. Smith & A. Jury (Eds.), *Workforce Development Theory and Practice in the Mental Health Sector* (pp. 1–35). Hershey, PA: IGI Global. doi:10.4018/978-1-5225-1874-7.ch001

Rodda, S. N., Abbott, M. W., Dowling, N. A., & Lubman, D. I. (2017). Workforce Development and E-Competency in Mental Health Services. In M. Smith & A. Jury (Eds.), *Workforce Development Theory and Practice in the Mental Health Sector* (pp. 284–301). Hershey, PA: IGI Global. doi:10.4018/978-1-5225-1874-7.ch014

Ruotsala, R. (2015). Networking around Supervisors in an Industrial Corporation. In T. Hansson (Ed.), *Contemporary Approaches to Activity Theory: Interdisciplinary Perspectives on Human Behavior* (pp. 198–213). Hershey, PA: IGI Global. doi:10.4018/978-1-4666-6603-0.ch012

Sandoval-Lucero, E., White, T. D., Haynes, D. E., Phillips, Q., Brame, J. D., & Sturtevant James, K. A. (2017). Engaging Inclusive Excellence: Creating a College With an Equity Mindset. In L. Leavitt, S. Wisdom, & K. Leavitt (Eds.), *Cultural Awareness and Competency Development in Higher Education* (pp. 40–60). Hershey, PA: IGI Global. doi:10.4018/978-1-5225-2145-7.ch003

Santhosh, K. R. (2016). Stress and Resilience in Parents of Intellectually Disabled Children. In R. Gopalan (Ed.), *Handbook of Research on Diagnosing, Treating, and Managing Intellectual Disabilities* (pp. 109–117). Hershey, PA: IGI Global. doi:10.4018/978-1-5225-0089-6.ch006

Sato, T., & Hodge, S. R. (2016). Asian International Graduate Students' Academic and Social Experiences in American Higher Education. In K. Bista & C. Foster (Eds.), *Exploring the Social and Academic Experiences of International Students in Higher Education Institutions* (pp. 1–20). Hershey, PA: IGI Global. doi:10.4018/978-1-4666-9749-2.ch001

Scupin, R. (2017). The Concept of Culture and Higher Education: An Anthropological Perspective. In L. Leavitt, S. Wisdom, & K. Leavitt (Eds.), *Cultural Awareness and Competency Development in Higher Education* (pp. 1–20). Hershey, PA: IGI Global. doi:10.4018/978-1-5225-2145-7.ch001

Seppänen, L., & Kloetzer, L. (2015). Micro-Analysis of Concepts for Developing Networking in Social Work. In T. Hansson (Ed.), *Contemporary Approaches to Activity Theory: Interdisciplinary Perspectives on Human Behavior* (pp. 162–180). Hershey, PA: IGI Global. doi:10.4018/978-1-4666-6603-0.ch010

Sertyesilisik, B. (2017). Enhancing Global Competency of Future Construction Professionals. In L. Leavitt, S. Wisdom, & K. Leavitt (Eds.), *Cultural Awareness and Competency Development in Higher Education* (pp. 272–287). Hershey, PA: IGI Global. doi:10.4018/978-1-5225-2145-7.ch016

Sharma, R., & Lohan, A. (2016). Psychosocial Interventions for Individuals with Intellectual Disability. In R. Gopalan (Ed.), *Handbook of Research on Diagnosing, Treating, and Managing Intellectual Disabilities* (pp. 262–282). Hershey, PA: IGI Global. doi:10.4018/978-1-5225-0089-6.ch014

Simuth, J. (2017). Psychological Impacts of Downsizing Trauma. In S. Hăša & R. Brunet-Thornton (Eds.), *Impact of Organizational Trauma on Workplace Behavior and Performance* (pp. 120–139). Hershey, PA: IGI Global. doi:10.4018/978-1-5225-2021-4.ch005

Sinha, P., Garg, A., Khanna, P., & Khanna, A. (2017). Management of Chronic Mental Illnesses and Substance Use Disorders. In B. Prasad (Ed.), *Chronic Mental Illness and the Changing Scope of Intervention Strategies, Diagnosis, and Treatment* (pp. 101–122). Hershey, PA: IGI Global. doi:10.4018/978-1-5225-0519-8.ch006

Smith, M., & Jury, A. F. (2017). Key Initiatives in New Zealand's Adult Mental Health Workforce Development. In M. Smith & A. Jury (Eds.), *Workforce Development Theory and Practice in the Mental Health Sector* (pp. 106–129). Hershey, PA: IGI Global. doi:10.4018/978-1-5225-1874-7.ch005

Sol, N. (2017). Fostering Intercultural Identity During Study Abroad to Strengthen Intercultural Competence. In L. Leavitt, S. Wisdom, & K. Leavitt (Eds.), *Cultural Awareness and Competency Development in Higher Education* (pp. 325–345). Hershey, PA: IGI Global. doi:10.4018/978-1-5225-2145-7.ch019

Soni, S. C. P., & Ahamed, P. C. (2017). Understanding and Management of Caregivers' Stress and Burden of Person with Obsessive Compulsive Disorder. In B. Prasad (Ed.), *Chronic Mental Illness and the Changing Scope of Intervention Strategies, Diagnosis, and Treatment* (pp. 124–142). Hershey, PA: IGI Global. doi:10.4018/978-1-5225-0519-8.ch007

Soria, K. M., & Lueck, S. M. (2016). High-Impact Educational Practices to Promote International Students' Engagement and Development: Evidence from Large, Public Research Universities. In K. Bista & C. Foster (Eds.), *Exploring the Social and Academic Experiences of International Students in Higher Education Institutions* (pp. 292–308). Hershey, PA: IGI Global. doi:10.4018/978-1-4666-9749-2.ch015

Srivastav, D., & Singh, T. B. (2017). Comorbidity Issues and Treatment in Chronic Mental Illness. In B. Prasad (Ed.), *Chronic Mental Illness and the Changing Scope of Intervention Strategies, Diagnosis, and Treatment* (pp. 77–100). Hershey, PA: IGI Global. doi:10.4018/978-1-5225-0519-8.ch005

St George, L. C., O'Hagan, M., Bradstreet, S., & Burge, M. (2017). The Emerging Field of Peer Support within Mental Health Services. In M. Smith & A. Jury (Eds.), *Workforce Development Theory and Practice in the Mental Health Sector* (pp. 222–250). Hershey, PA: IGI Global. doi:10.4018/978-1-5225-1874-7.ch011

Starr-Glass, D. (2017). Can Higher Education Really Produce Global Citizens?: Self-Identification and Architectures of Mobility. In L. Leavitt, S. Wisdom, & K. Leavitt (Eds.), *Cultural Awareness and Competency Development in Higher Education* (pp. 304–324). Hershey, PA: IGI Global. doi:10.4018/978-1-5225-2145-7.ch018

Szymanski, M., & Schindler, E. (2017). Embracing Organizational Trauma: Positive Effects of Death Experiences on Organizational Culture – Three Short Case Studies. In S. Háša & R. Brunet-Thornton (Eds.), *Impact of Organizational Trauma on Workplace Behavior and Performance* (pp. 247–263). Hershey, PA: IGI Global. doi:10.4018/978-1-5225-2021-4.ch010

Tavaragi, M. S. (2017). Chronic Mental Illness in Prisons: Global Scenario. In B. Prasad (Ed.), *Chronic Mental Illness and the Changing Scope of Intervention Strategies, Diagnosis, and Treatment* (pp. 203–224). Hershey, PA: IGI Global. doi:10.4018/978-1-5225-0519-8.ch011

Tavaragi, M. S., & C., S. (2017). Global Burden of Mental Disorders: Quality of Care and Unmet Needs for Treatment of Chronic Mental Illness. In B. Prasad (Ed.), *Chronic Mental Illness and the Changing Scope of Intervention Strategies, Diagnosis, and Treatment* (pp. 164-186). Hershey, PA: IGI Global. doi:10.4018/978-1-5225-0519-8.ch009

Tekin, A. K. (2016). Parent Involvement in the Education of Children with Chronic Diseases: Working and Sharing for Children. In M. Gordon (Ed.), *Challenges Surrounding the Education of Children with Chronic Diseases* (pp. 151–164). Hershey, PA: IGI Global. doi:10.4018/978-1-4666-9452-1.ch008

Toiviainen, H. (2015). Interventions for Learning at Global Workplaces. In T. Hansson (Ed.), *Contemporary Approaches to Activity Theory: Interdisciplinary Perspectives on Human Behavior* (pp. 214–227). Hershey, PA: IGI Global. doi:10.4018/978-1-4666-6603-0.ch013

Tran, B. (2017). Impact of Organizational Trauma on Workplace Behavior and Performance: Workplace Bullying Due to (In)Competency. In S. Háša, & R. Brunet-Thornton (Eds.), Impact of Organizational Trauma on Workplace Behavior and Performance (pp. 221-245). Hershey, PA: IGI Global. doi:10.4018/978-1-5225-2021-4.ch009

Tripathi, M. A., & Sridevi, G. (2017). Psychotherapeutic Interventions in Emotional and Behavioural Problems with Adolescents. In B. Prasad (Ed.), *Chronic Mental Illness and the Changing Scope of Intervention Strategies, Diagnosis, and Treatment* (pp. 321–333). Hershey, PA: IGI Global. doi:10.4018/978-1-5225-0519-8.ch018

Tseng, M., & Pluta, R. M. (2016). Educating Students with Chronic Illness: How the Old Service Model Fails. In M. Gordon (Ed.), *Challenges Surrounding the Education of Children with Chronic Diseases* (pp. 227–246). Hershey, PA: IGI Global. doi:10.4018/978-1-4666-9452-1.ch011

Vaccaro, A., D'Aloisio, B., Hoyt, T., Chartelain, A., Croft, S. D., & Stevens, B. (2017). Developing Social Justice and Inclusion Competencies Through Semi-Structured Reflection Papers. In L. Leavitt, S. Wisdom, & K. Leavitt (Eds.), *Cultural Awareness and Competency Development in Higher Education* (pp. 75–91). Hershey, PA: IGI Global. doi:10.4018/978-1-5225-2145-7.ch005

Vora, K. S. (2016). Family Members as Caregivers of Individuals with Intellectual Disabilities: Caregiving for Individuals with Intellectual Disabilities. In R. Gopalan (Ed.), *Handbook of Research on Diagnosing, Treating, and Managing Intellectual Disabilities* (pp. 118–138). Hershey, PA: IGI Global. doi:10.4018/978-1-5225-0089-6.ch007

Vorkapić, S. T. (2017). *Measuring the Psychological and Electrophysiological Attributes of Human Personality: Emerging Research and Opportunities* (pp. 1–242). Hershey, PA: IGI Global. doi:10.4018/978-1-5225-2283-6

Watson, A. L. (2017). Developing a Practice of Cultural Awareness in Pre-Service Teachers by Promoting Positive Dialogue Around Diversity. In L. Leavitt, S. Wisdom, & K. Leavitt (Eds.), *Cultural Awareness and Competency Development in Higher Education* (pp. 223–236). Hershey, PA: IGI Global. doi:10.4018/978-1-5225-2145-7.ch013

Watts, L., & Gullberg, B. (2015). Acculturation Processes and Expatriate Behavior. In T. Hansson (Ed.), *Contemporary Approaches to Activity Theory: Interdisciplinary Perspectives on Human Behavior* (pp. 285–303). Hershey, PA: IGI Global. doi:10.4018/978-1-4666-6603-0.ch017

Williams, G. M., & Case, R. E. (2016). When in Rome: Socializing International Teaching Assistants into the US Higher Education Norms. In K. Bista & C. Foster (Eds.), *Exploring the Social and Academic Experiences of International Students in Higher Education Institutions* (pp. 156–174). Hershey, PA: IGI Global. doi:10.4018/978-1-4666-9749-2.ch009

Wilson, K. B., Pitt, J. S., Raheem, M. A., Acklin, C. L., & Wilson, J. M. (2017). Multicultural Counseling Competencies: Why Is It Difficult to Apply What We Know…? In L. Leavitt, S. Wisdom, & K. Leavitt (Eds.), *Cultural Awareness and Competency Development in Higher Education* (pp. 237–254). Hershey, PA: IGI Global. doi:10.4018/978-1-5225-2145-7.ch014

Woodend, J., Nutter, S., Lei, D., & Cairns, S. (2016). Exploring the Experiences of International Students' Partners: Implications for the Post-Secondary Context. In K. Bista & C. Foster (Eds.), *Exploring the Social and Academic Experiences of International Students in Higher Education Institutions* (pp. 96–114). Hershey, PA: IGI Global. doi:10.4018/978-1-4666-9749-2.ch006

Wright, M. F. (2016). School Bullying and Students with Intellectual Disabilities. In R. Gopalan (Ed.), *Handbook of Research on Diagnosing, Treating, and Managing Intellectual Disabilities* (pp. 33–53). Hershey, PA: IGI Global. doi:10.4018/978-1-5225-0089-6.ch003

Yu, X., Isensee, E., & Kappler, B. (2016). Using Data Wisely to Improve International Student Satisfaction: Insights Gained from International Student Barometer. In K. Bista & C. Foster (Eds.), *Exploring the Social and Academic Experiences of International Students in Higher Education Institutions* (pp. 212–232). Hershey, PA: IGI Global. doi:10.4018/978-1-4666-9749-2.ch012

Zhao, J. (2015). Project-Based Instruction in Teaching Chinese as a Foreign Language. In T. Hansson (Ed.), *Contemporary Approaches to Activity Theory: Interdisciplinary Perspectives on Human Behavior* (pp. 108–127). Hershey, PA: IGI Global. doi:10.4018/978-1-4666-6603-0.ch007

Zhao, J., & Ng, D. F. (2016). Understanding Language Experiences of International ESL Students in U.S. Classrooms. In K. Bista & C. Foster (Eds.), *Exploring the Social and Academic Experiences of International Students in Higher Education Institutions* (pp. 175–196). Hershey, PA: IGI Global. doi:10.4018/978-1-4666-9749-2.ch010

Zhou, W., & Austin, S. (2017). Developing Intercultural Awareness Within Teacher Preparation Program. In L. Leavitt, S. Wisdom, & K. Leavitt (Eds.), *Cultural Awareness and Competency Development in Higher Education* (pp. 189–206). Hershey, PA: IGI Global. doi:10.4018/978-1-5225-2145-7.ch011

About the Authors

Melissa Martin, Ph.D., is an Assistant Professor in the Teacher Education department at the State University of New York (SUNY) – Plattsburgh. Currently, she teaches courses related to Childhood Education and Special Education to preservice general and special educators. Previously, she was a self-contained special education teacher at an elementary school in South Carolina for several years. Her research interests include writing instruction and motivation for students with disabilities and collaboration and co-teaching in higher education.

Jean Mockry, CAS and MS Ed, is a Lecturer and Program Leader in the Undergraduate Childhood Education at the State University of New York at Plattsburgh, in Plattsburgh, NY. She earned these degrees from SUNY Plattsburgh with her MS Ed thesis focus on comparing elementary reading instructional programs and her CAS thesis an analysis of eating disorders in High School students. She has been a practitioner for over twenty years in teaching elementary students and high school students English, along with serving as school counselor to both elementary and high school students and administration as a building principal (K-8). For the last decade she has worked in Higher Education as a Lecturer and student teaching supervisor in Teacher Education in both the undergraduate and graduate programs. She carries a strong interest in teacher preparation and in mental health.

Alison Puliatte, Ph.D., is an Assistant Professor of Teacher Education at the State University of New York at Plattsburgh. She earned a Ph.D. in Educational Psychology with a concentration in Learning, Development and Instruction from the CUNY Graduate Center. She earned a C.A.S. in Educational Leadership, an M.S.Ed. in Special Education, and a B.A. in Psychology and Elementary Education from Queens College, CUNY. She was an elementary teacher in Nassau County, NY where she taught prekindergarten, first and fifth grade in an integrated co-teaching setting. She served as an elementary school principal for 12 years in Lynbrook, NY. She currently teaches undergraduate and graduate courses in Childhood and Special Education. Her research areas of interest include teacher knowledge, literacy, social contexts, and teacher perceptions.

Denise Simard, Ph.D., is presently an Associate Professor and Interim Dean of the School of Education, Health, and Human Services at the State University of New York at Plattsburgh, in Plattsburgh NY. She began her professional journey as a special education teacher. She then began collaborating with children and families to access technology devices and services to empower them to be more independent in their daily lives. She used those experiences to become an advocate for change and subsequently managed local and state professional development initiatives related to the infusion of technology into instructional practices to improve learning outcomes for all students, especially those with special needs. She also supported the strategic planning process, facilitation, and evaluation of online learning communities for education organizations on a local, state, and national level. Currently she teaches undergraduate classes in the childhood education program and graduate classes in special education. Her areas of interest and research include multiculturalism, special education, assistive technology, online learning, and communities of practice. Through her various roles in higher education, she has had the wonderful opportunity to examine aspects of leadership and the nuances and intricacies involved.

Maureen E. Squires, Ed.D., is an Associate Professor of Teacher Education, Department Chair, and member of the Center for Teaching Excellence Task Force at the State University of New York at Plattsburgh, in Plattsburgh, N.Y. She earned an Ed.D. in Educational Theory and Practice (2011) and a C.A.S. in Educational Leadership (2008) from Binghamton University, an M.S.Ed. in Special Education (2003) from LeMoyne College, and a B.A. in English (2001) with a concentration in Secondary Education from Nazareth College. She holds multiple New York State teaching and leadership certifications. Her professional career began as an English teacher at LaFayette Junior/Senior High School in LaFayette, N.Y. Currently, she teaches graduate courses and supervises teacher candidate fieldwork in the Special Education program and the Adolescence Education program. Her areas of interest and research include teacher preparation, special education, ethics and education, and the education of Native Americans/American Indians.

Index

K

M

N

P

R

S

T

U

CPSIA information can be obtained
at www.ICGtesting.com
Printed in the USA
BVHW010039160120
568897BV00012B/31/P

9 781522 537939